Medicine's
Dilemmas

Medicine's Dilemmas

Infinite Needs
versus
Finite Resources

WILLIAM L. KISSICK, M.D., Dr. P.H.

To Mitzi and George —
professor and mentor
and leader.
Bill Kissick

YALE UNIVERSITY PRESS
NEW HAVEN AND LONDON

Set in Janson type by The Composing Room of Michigan, Inc., Grand
Rapids, Michigan. Printed in the United States of America by Vail-Ballou
Press, Binghamton, New York.

Library of Congress Cataloging-in-Publication Data

Kissick, William L.
Medicine's dilemmas : infinite needs versus finite resources / William L.
Kissick.
p. cm. — (A Yale fastback)
Includes bibliographical references and index.
ISBN 0-300-05964-7 (cloth : alk. paper). — ISBN 0-300-05965-5 (pbk. : alk.
paper)
1. Medical care—United States—Cost control.   2. Medical policy—
United States.   3. Medical economics—United States.   I. Title.
II. Series.
[DNLM: 1. Delivery of Health Care—United States.   2. Public Policy—
United States.   3. Insurance, Health—United States.   W 84 AA1 K58m
1994]
RA410.53.K55   1994
338.4'73621'0973—dc20
DNLM/DLC
for Library of Congress   94-1137 CIP

A catalogue record for this book is available from the British Library.

The paper in this book meets the guidelines for permanence and durability
of the Committee on Production Guidelines for Book Longevity of the
Council on Library Resources.

10   9   8   7   6   5   4   3   2   1

To
Joan Kuprevich
Colleague and Friend

Contents

List of Figures

List of Tables

Preface

Midway through the first hundred days of the Clinton administration, Louis Harris testified to the House Select Committee on Aging about a nationwide poll on health care that he had conducted shortly before the inauguration. He concluded that "first, they [Americans] want quality health care, which will cover a wide range of services. Second, they want everyone in the nation, without exception, covered for proper health care. Third, they want what they feel are the widely spiraling costs of health care brought under control. And fourth, they want to be able to choose their own doctors and hospitals and they want those physicians and hospitals to be mainly controlled by the private sector." The results of the poll laid out an ambitious agenda for the reform of health care in our society. A health-care task force of five hundred, chaired by Hillary Rodham Clinton, took up the challenge.

Three decades earlier, in April 1964, President Lyndon B. Johnson had appointed an eight-person White House task force on health. As one of three staff members, I participated in the genesis of the Great

Society health programs that were revealed to the Congress in the president's health message on 7 January 1965. The lead proposal was the hospital insurance for the elderly that would become Medicare. Of some two dozen program and budgetary authorizations recommended, the Eighty-ninth Congress, which deliberated throughout 1965 and 1966, enacted virtually every one.

Late one night in December 1964 when we were drafting the president's health message, Wilbur Cohen, assistant secretary of legislation in the Department of Health, Education, and Welfare and the principal architect of Medicare, said to me, "Bill, never forget—health policy is 10 percent legislation and 90 percent implementation." As I await the legislation of health-care reform in the 1990s, I am concerned about the mechanisms for implementation into the twenty-first century.

For the past quarter-century, I have sought to understand the effects of the Great Society's health legislation, along with subsequent initiatives of the Nixon, Ford, Carter, Reagan, and Bush administrations. As a professor in the School of Medicine and the Wharton School at the University of Pennsylvania, I have attempted to explain to my students the endeavor that accounts for one-seventh of our total economy, the American health-care enterprise.

When I arrived at Penn in 1968, my colleagues in the School of Medicine told me, "No cost is too great to save a life or treat disease." Across the campus, my colleagues in the Wharton School cautioned, "Resources are limited and choices must be made." Since 1968 I have been crossing the street separating the medical school and the Wharton School almost daily in search of strategies for addressing the dilemmas these two views create.

My travels around the country speaking to audiences of hospital trustees, physicians, health-care executives, nurses, other health-care professionals, and consumer groups have helped me appreciate the convictions expressed in the Harris poll. Most Americans are convinced that we enjoy the finest health care in the world. If by that we mean that our finest is unexcelled anywhere in the world, the conviction is accurate. If, however, we imply that all Americans have access to the finest health care, then we believe in a myth.

I was raised in the automotive capital of the world, where my father worked for U.S. Rubber, a major supplier for General Motors; his younger brother worked for the Ford Motor Company and his sister's husband for Chrysler. Thanksgiving dinners resembled a meeting of the Big Three. My father and my uncles discussed new models, production runs, marketing strategies, and sales. As a child, I thought the Detroit automotive companies were giants that strode the world in seven-league boots. In the 1950s, they were indeed forces as compelling in our nation's economy as health care is today.

In those years, as I attended college and medical school, I spent my summers working construction jobs in the Detroit area. While Ford and General Motors helped finance my higher education, I helped build a Lincoln-Mercury assembly plant and the General Motors Technical Center. My colleagues were carpenters, laborers, rod busters, plumbers, pipe fitters, electricians, and ironworkers. When they found out that I was a medical student, they questioned me about every problem they had ever encountered with a physician or a hospital.

My colleagues taught me valuable lessons. Patients may lack information, but they don't lack interest. They have far more interest in maintaining their cars, however, than in maintaining their bodies. They damn physicians and hospitals in general but consider their own physicians virtual saints. This disregard of personal responsibility for one's own health, coupled with ambivalence about the health-care system, underlies any discussion of health-care reform at the threshold of the twenty-first century.

The Detroit auto industry played a major role in the development and growth of third-party health insurance during World War II. The arsenal of democracy, as Detroit was known, negotiated generous fringe benefits for health insurance at a time when defense contracts were on a cost-plus basis and wages were controlled. Both labor and management benefited, as the War Department picked up the tab. By 1976, Blue Cross and Blue Shield had grown to be the largest single supplier for General Motors, and Metropolitan Life Insurance, covering workers' compensation, was second; U.S. Steel was third. Today corporate America is experiencing a crisis in health-care costs.

As I look back over the experiences of my youth and those of my professional career, I see many parallels between the Detroit auto industry and the American health-care enterprise. The latter has three times the revenues and eight times the labor force of the former and virtually all its problems. Health care today hardly resembles a well-engineered, fuel-efficient, compact, cost-effective, smooth-handling vehicle that will get us where we need to go at an affordable price. How long will it take for hospital trustees, physicians, nurses, and health-care managers to appreciate the imperatives of significant change, the message that the American auto industry chose to ignore for so long? Would that the restructuring of health care could be less disruptive and painful than that of the American auto industry.

In these pages I have sought to reconcile the goals of the health sciences with those of the management sciences. George G. Lundberg, the editor of the *Journal of the American Medical Association*, has warned of the danger of a "health-care meltdown," but the health professions have been joined by corporate America and the electorate in an effort to avoid such a disaster. In reviewing the crises and the alternatives, I hope I have laid out the requirements for long-term strategies.

Acknowledgments

Health policy is made by, as well as for, people—a multitude of people. Like health policy, this book has had many collaborators. A number of individuals have influenced my thinking, some in little more than a brief encounter. While literature is cited, people are often quoted or paraphrased anonymously.

Medicine's Dilemmas is a personal statement on health policy. As such, it reflects a professional experience spanning three decades and owes much to all who have shared in that experience. The Oath of Hippocrates admonishes me, as it does all physicians, "to reckon him who taught me this Art equally dear to me as my parents." Many of my teachers are like family. Five stand out as mentors as well as teachers: the late John Devereaux Thompson, professor of health services administration at the Yale University School of Public Health; George A. Silver, chief of the Division of Social Medicine at the Montefiore Hospital Medical Center and deputy assistant secretary for health (1966–68); William H. Stewart, surgeon general of the United States (1965–69); Sir George Godber, chief medical officer of the British National Health Service (1960–73); and Samuel P. Martin III, professor emeritus of medicine and health-care management at the University of Pennsylvania. Although I now mentor young physicians, nurses, and health-care managers, I continue a relationship with my own mentors. During the writing of this book they provided inspiration, criticism, and counsel.

I began my work in 1986, during a sabbatical spent studying health-policy research and educational programs for the Pew Charitable Trusts. The entrée and financial support provided by the foundation enabled me to visit, and test ideas with, leading authorities on health policy in the United States. My thanks to Rebecca Rimel, president of the Pew Charitable Trusts, and Thomas Langfitt, president of the Glenmede Trust.

The late Robert D. Eilers, founding executive director of the Leonard Davis Institute of Health Economics, was instrumental in recruiting me to the University of Pennsylvania. The institute, whose governing board I now chair, was endowed in 1967 by Leonard and Sophie Davis. Their vision launched a preeminent interdisciplinary endeavor in health-services research and health policy. I consider them benefactors of this work.

Most books I have read acknowledge the inspiration and role of key individuals in the author's life. My wife, Priscilla, and our children—William, Robert-John, Jonathan, and Elizabeth—have provided well-meaning critical insight over the years. I have promised to share the royalties after deducting reimbursement of tuition expenses.

A number of students have served as research assistants on ad hoc assignments. Since their monetary compensation has been small, they are herewith gratefully acknowledged: Terrance Akin, Cynthia Armstrong, Rebecca Baxt, Anna Buckingham, Elizabeth Burgess, Christopher Cameron, Christopher Dowdell, Jacqueline Einstein, Cam Enarson, Joel Forkosch, Roseann Jones, Risa Mathisson, Amy Raslevich, Mark Rogers, Diane Schretzman, and Robert Stebbins. A special thanks to Linda Bornyasz for her dedication. Graphics were designed by GRAPHICAE of Philadelphia and Steve Keller of Graphic Arts of Lakewood in Golden, Colorado.

The several drafts of this book had a multitude of readers, whose dedication in reviewing chapters, not to mention a narrative that reached 130,000 words at one point, brings new meaning to collegial friendship. My thanks to Sandy Barth, Bernie Bloom, Bill Bluemle, Bruce Bradley, Timothy Brewer, Richmond Brown, Anna-Marie Chirico, Patricia Danzon, Stanley Flink, John Freymann, Virginia Froman, Eli Ginzberg, Clifford Graham, Christine Grant, Robert Hess, Bill Hiscock, Chuck Honaker, Ted Huth, Ted Loder, Mary McGeein, Sandy Norman, John O'Donnell, Perry Pepper, Douglas Peters, David Smith, Nick Spinelli, and Howard Spiro.

Three colleagues—Tony Kovner, Shep Nuland, and Bill Stewart—have my extensive gratitude. They demonstrated rare commitment and forbearance, reading and analyzing the entire manuscript several times. I hope they conclude that I finally got it right.

While authors attempt to write manuscripts, editors create published books. Gae Holladay patiently taught me the imperatives of audience, voice, and advocacy. She sought to identify and eliminate all excess words while getting the rest of them in the right order. I've learned that editing is the essence of life.

I was fortunate to have the counsel of professionals in the world of publishing. I wish to thank Donald Lamm of Norton, Tom Rotell and Patricia Smith of the University of Pennsylvania Press, and John Ryden and Jean Thomson Black of Yale University Press. They made this publication a reality.

As a medical student I often sought solitude and contemplation in the Yale Medical Historical Library. The stuffed easy chairs and sofas gave rest to the body as one sought to nurture the mind. Books intended as diversionary reading were displayed on the end tables. The distinctive bookplates read, "Those they praise, but these they read." I hope this book is read by many diverse stakeholders in health care. To paraphrase Georges Clemenceau, himself a physician, health care is too important to be left to the providers.

Chapter 1
Somebody Has to Pay

Everyone deserves the finest health care.

In 1955, during his first term, President Dwight D. Eisenhower suffered a heart attack—more precisely, an acute myocardial infarction. Paul Dudley White, professor of medicine at the Harvard Medical School and the leading cardiologist in the nation, was summoned to the president's bedside at the Fitzsimmons Army Medical Center.[1] Dr. White supervised the most advanced therapy: bedrest, oxygen, digoxin to strengthen cardiac contractions, anticoagulants to thin the blood and to prevent further clotting, and morphine for pain.

That year, as a third-year medical student, I participated in the treatment of another patient who had suffered a myocardial infarction. This patient was ten years younger than the president, but our therapy was much the same. At the time, we could afford to administer the same treatment as the nation's first patient received to every other patient with a heart attack.

Two decades after President Eisenhower's heart attack, Judge Arnold Bucher of Lancaster County, Pennsylvania, only fifty miles from

President Eisenhower's farm in Gettysburg, also underwent treatment for heart disease.[2] His therapy was vastly different from Eisenhower's: the judge had two coronary artery bypass grafts. Since the technology was introduced in the 1970s, millions of these procedures have been performed, representing only one of the biomedical advances for treating heart disease in the decades since bedrest, oxygen, digoxin, anticoagulants, and morphine were prescribed for President Eisenhower. Present diagnosis and treatment include angiocardiography, streptokinase, tissue plasminogen activator, and transluminal balloon angioplasty. More than twenty innovations have been introduced in cardiology in the past two decades alone.[3]

Perhaps even more dramatic than advances in heart-disease therapies are advances in information technology.[4] Computerized axial tomography (CAT scanning), magnetic resonance imaging (MRI), proton emission tomography (PET scan), and sophisticated technologies in the clinical laboratory tell more about patients than doctors can always effectively use. The extraordinary capacity of the medical establishment to identify and measure human deficiencies and to develop technologies to treat them complements the physician's conviction that no cost is too great to save a life. But who is going to pay?

The golden rule of health care in our society is that everyone deserves the finest health care attainable, provided someone else pays. But in what I call the iron triangle of health care (fig. 1), access, quality, and cost containment have equal angles, representing identical priorities, and an expansion of any one angle compromises one or both of the other two. All societies confront the equal tensions among access to health services, quality of health care, and cost containment. Tradeoffs are inevitable regardless of the size of the triangle. Call them resource allocation or rationing, they are choices our society must make.

In recent decades we have expanded both access and quality, but only through substantial increases in costs. During the 1980s, competition in health affairs was the preferred mechanism for obtaining value in health services, but cost containment on the part of government, third-party carriers, and employers has affected quality, as well as access. Some proposals for national health insurance argue that access

Cost Containment

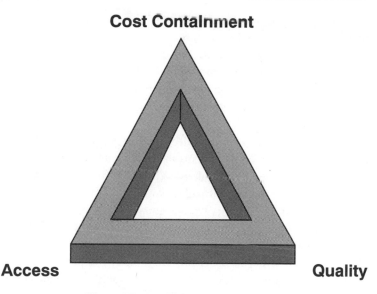

Access   Quality

Fig. 1. The Iron Triangle of Health Care

can be expanded to include the entire population at reduced costs. Such a scheme would require dramatic modifications in the quality of health care as we know it.

How costs are allocated among beneficiaries and kinds of services is often the major concern when cost containment is discussed. Most proposals for national health insurance make cost containment the lead issue, or at least a prominent one. Everyone's prime targets are waste, fraud, and abuse, but few proposals offer specifics. Administrative expenses, estimated at 24 percent of expenditures, are another target for cost cutting.[5] The Canadian system seeks to cut administrative costs by eliminating insurance companies as third-party carriers and substituting government as the single payer.

Health care in America consumes 14 percent of the gross domestic product, yet some 40 million citizens are uninsured. A health policy that guarantees access for everyone in the population is ultimately a tax policy. Who, though, is to be taxed and by what mechanisms? Once citizens and legislators accept the link between access and taxation, the debate shifts to the way various forms of taxation affect the economy.

Cost-effectiveness is often championed as a solution to the problem of the iron triangle of health care. It seems to deliver appropriate quality at the lowest unit cost. But the addition of universal access returns one to the question of trade-offs. Although it may be politically unattractive, a health-care strategy must balance cost with quality and access to yield the greatest good for the greatest number.

Biomedical advances in recent decades have given us the capacity to do more for 260 million Americans than our society can afford to do. Biomedical and science technology so dominate medicine of the late twentieth century that it is difficult to appreciate that they were virtually nonexistent at the turn of the century. Lawrence Henderson of Harvard is credited with the observation that not until 1911 did the average patient consulting the average physician at random have a better than fifty-fifty chance of benefiting from the encounter. Until then, the general practitioner's bag contained vials of pills, herbs, and elixirs; assorted surgical instruments; a spring scale; and prescription sheets. A physician today would require an eighteen-wheel semitrailer to haul all the tools of modern medicine—the clinical laboratory, imaging technology, and personnel.

Medicine has built a century of scientific and technological achievement on two dozen centuries of tradition, beginning in 1890 with the development of a diphtheria antitoxin (table 1). Wilhelm Konrad Röntgen introduced X rays in 1895 as the first marvel of imaging. The work of Frederick Grant Banting and Charles Herbert Best at the University of Toronto in 1922 brought forth insulin for the treatment of diabetes. Sulfonamides in the 1930s and penicillin in the 1940s, followed by broad-spectrum antibiotics in the 1950s, gave medical practice the power to cure as well as to care. Organ transplants began in 1954 at the Peter Bent Brigham Hospital in Boston, where the kidney of one identical twin was implanted in the other. Less than a decade later, artificial renal dialysis was developed for the treatment of chronic end-stage kidney disease. The pump oxygenator (heart-lung machine) sustains hundreds of thousands of open-heart procedures each year, and the artificial heart has been implanted experimentally. Meanwhile, CAT and MRI imaging has brought new dimensions to diagnosis. In 1953 James Watson and Francis Crick launched molecu-

Table 1
A Century of Biomedical Science and Technology

Diphtheria antitoxin	1890
X ray	1895
Insulin	1922
Penicillin	1942
Broad-spectrum antibiotics	1950
Double helix	1953
Kidney transplantation	1954
Polio vaccine	1958
Chronic renal dialysis	1962
Open-heart surgery	1970
CAT scanning	1972
Jarvik 7 artificial heart	1982
Gene therapy	1990

lar biology at the Cavendish Laboratories at Cambridge University when they revealed the structure of the double helix. Their research led to molecular medicine and to the advent of gene therapy at the National Institutes of Health in 1990. These are but highlights from a cornucopia of scientific advances.

Biomedical research and development since World War II is a societal phenomenon. It has been estimated that 90 percent of the biomedical scientists in the history of the world are working in laboratories at present. Recent scientific insights into the etiology and pathogenesis of Acquired Immune Deficiency Syndrome (AIDS) illustrates the potential of the scientific enterprise, spurred by worldwide competition and collaboration, for the development of new knowledge.

Still, the relentless tensions of the iron triangle intrude. The biomedical advances and technological innovations shown in figure 2 are illustrative of the many that have occurred since I entered medical school in 1953. Three—polio vaccine, gene therapy, and chronic renal dialysis—dramatize differences. The model for biomedical aspirations could be termed the polio paradigm, as polio vaccine has the highest cost-benefit ratio of any postwar biomedical development. When the benefits in lives saved, disability prevented, or net present value of future income are measured against the costs of research,

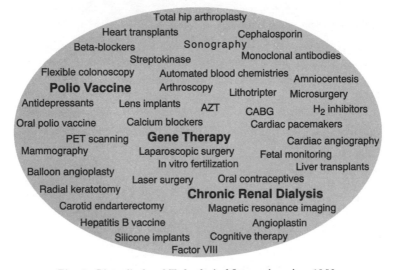

Fig. 2. Biomedical and Technological Innovations since 1953

production, and distribution, the payoffs are extraordinary. Chronic renal dialysis, by contrast, represents intermediate technology that does not offer prevention or cure but sustains life of diminished quality at high cost, in this instance $30,000 to $35,000 per year. Although gene therapy aspires to prevent and cure, the polio paradigm has thus far set a standard impossible to meet.

The miracles of modern medicine, from organ transplants to magnetic resonance imaging, raise troubling issues. One is the realization that the availability of a treatment is not the same as its accessibility to the general population. If there is to be equal access, somebody has to pay.

Health-care finance was different at the beginning of the century, when Samuel P. Martin, Jr., a general practitioner in East Prairie, Missouri, used a barter and modified fee system in his practice. A wooden box in the waiting room in his office indicated to his patients that some form of payment was expected for his services. The size and character of that compensation was left to the individual patient, but the values and ethics of the small community required that appropriate payment be made. Moreover, the physician had a fairly good notion of each patient's economic status.

The fee system has prevailed, but with the physician determining the size of the fee and the volume of services. Fees are a powerful incentive for services. The larger the fees a patient offers for medical care, the greater the physician's incentive to provide those services. For many years the financing of health care remained relatively simple: patients, when able, paid physicians out of pocket, in cash or in kind. The ethics of medicine required in turn that the physician respond regardless of the patient's ability to pay.

Other mechanisms of compensating physicians emerged. Large group practices such as those at the Mayo Clinic and the Cleveland Clinic collected fees from patients but paid salaries—fee for time   to the physician partners. Prepaid group practices such as Kaiser Permanente used capitation—fee per patient per unit time. Fee for service, salary, and capitation each have relative advantages and disadvantages for the patient, the physician, and the community. Recognizing this, the British National Health Service uses all three mechanisms for compensating the general practitioner

Paying the hospital took a different tack, as illustrated by the system established by the Pennsylvania Hospital, the nation's first, founded by Ben Franklin in 1751.[6] Its services were provided as a charitable contribution by Philadelphia's wealthiest families. The rich themselves, of course, would not have thought to use the Pennsylvania Hospital; they would have been treated in their homes by private physicians. Hospitals were for the less fortunate.

Contemporary hospital financing began in Dallas in 1929.[7] Schoolteachers concerned about the cost of hospital care struck a bargain with the Baylor University Hospital. They made prepayments to the hospital—fifty cents per teacher per month—literally deposits in exchange for the commitment of hospital services if and when needed. Thus the forerunner of Blue Cross was launched. Over time, retrospective cost-based reimbursement for hospitals became the equivalent of fee for service to the physician. In both instances, third parties were increasingly expected to pay for all services prescribed by physicians, provided by hospitals, and used by patients. The complexity of hospital finance is, of course, enormous, involving institutions with thousands of employees, payrolls totaling hundreds of millions of dollars, volumes of services measured in hundreds of thousands of patient days, capital assets in the hundreds of millions—and community mandates to provide free care.[8]

To cover those patients with no coverage (the so-called bad debts), third-party insurance of all types has to be juggled with the time-honored tradition of cross-subsidization. While no one expects a store to provide goods and services without receiving payment, hospitals and physicians are expected to do just that. Citizens demand the service when they have or feel the need. In assuming health care is a right, they ignore the economist's first principle—there's no such thing as a free lunch. Health care cannot be free. Somebody has to pay. That somebody is all of us.

When Lyndon Johnson signed the legislation enacting Medicare in 1965, many considered the plan for the elderly a precedent for the rest of the population. Although Medicare was a herculean political achievement, requiring the efforts of two presidents, it lacked innovation and precluded restructuring of health services; in retrospect, indeed, it seems a modest accomplishment. Using tax dollars, Medicare replicated the open-ended financing of Blue Cross and Blue Shield, thirty-year-old concepts, for only 10 percent of the population. But technology, utilization, and the role of demography were underestimated. Since 1965, Medicare has authorized expenditures of hundreds of billions of dollars into a health-care economy undisciplined by markets, adequate regulation, or public ownership and operation.

The combination of extraordinary biomedical advances and national health insurance for the elderly gave society false confidence in the ability of its therapeutic and financial resources to meet health-care needs. Paradoxically, these advances and increased government financing led us to our present dilemmas. Technologies create need as well as respond to it, and unconstrained third-party reimbursement stimulates health-care utilization.

In seven seasons on prime-time television, Marcus Welby, M.D., never missed a diagnosis, had time for every patient, mentored a young colleague, was always compassionate, was never sued for malpractice, and supported himself on one patient per week. He practiced in the second decade of Medicare and could refer patients for organ transplants, artificial hips, and chronic renal dialysis. Health-care expenditures were increasing at 12 to 18 percent per year. It was not Utopia, but on balance times were pretty good.

The Marcus Welby scenario symbolized the aspirations of organized medicine:

Authority, Autonomy, and Prerogative. Medicine is an archetypical profession, enjoying extraordinary authority, autonomy, and prerogative.[9] Public opinion polls in the 1950s and 1960s showed physicians to be as highly esteemed as Supreme Court justices. Society has granted medical personnel control over a body of knowledge, its transmission, and its application. The patient places trust in physicians as advocates and healers.

Free Choice of Physician, Fee for Service, and Solo Practice. As Medicare was being drafted, the American Medical Association proclaimed that the sovereignty of the profession of medicine required free choice of physician, fee for service, and solo practice. Among some physicians, these conditions of practice bordered on religious conviction.

Usual, Customary, and Reasonable Fees. The advent of Blue Shield in th 1930s brought fee schedules for surgical procedures. Procedures were of course easier to count and measure than medical therapy was. Medicare Part B ratified the concept of reimbursement of fees that were usual, customary, and reasonable.

Physician's Markets. A shortage of physicians in the 1950s and 1960s contributed to a classic seller's market in which demand for services far exceeded supply. Establishing a practice required little more than hanging out a shingle.

Voluntary Hospital Staffs. Many physician services are highly dependent on hospitals. The privilege of using a hospital's services and relying on its nursing care is achieved by belonging to the hospital's voluntary staff. In many communities a physician may serve on the voluntary staffs of two or more hospitals.

Retrospective Cost-Based Reimbursement. The principle that has guided hospital financing for decades can be summarized as follows: provide the care, determine the cost, and be reimbursed by third-party insurance companies such as Blue Cross. It is the equivalent of giving a credit card to a young adult and saying, "I will reimburse all your expenditures on a monthly basis." The young adult goes to a store and says, "Give me what you think I need."

The Marcus Welby scenario and the demands of medical professionals helped escalate health-care spending to almost twice that of any of the country's competitors in world markets.[10] While reform is imperative, there is no quick fix. The next chapter surveys the achievements that have been made in health care and some of the challenges that remain.

Chapter 2
Health-Care Issues
of the 1990s

There will always be
ten leading causes of death.

Most of the health-care issues of the 1990s will no doubt be with us in the next century as well. Even if the medical establishment solves the ten current top issues, there will be new challenges. As Sir Geoffrey Vickers observes, "The history of public health can be written as a constant redefinition of the unacceptable."[1] Many of the issues that concern us today will be displaced by emerging priorities and intensifying crises.

It is virtually impossible to find a social institution in the United States that does not affect the health-care enterprise or is not influenced by it. Decisions concerning taxes, agricultural subsidies, the highway speed limit, minimum wages, and educational investments all touch the enterprise to varying degrees. Health care draws on a diffuse and intricate knowledge base. The efforts of molecular biologists to map the human genome currently occupy the limelight. But the economist, political scientist, and ethicist stand poised to capture the stage of health affairs in the twenty-first century. What are some of

11

the issues faced by health-care consumers and providers and the population at large?

Health-Care Costs

In a survey I conducted for a major foundation, I asked more than one hundred respondents, all prominent in health affairs, to itemize the probable leading health-care issues for the 1990s.[2] Most respondents identified cost containment as the major issue. One respondent identified three leading issues: (1) health-care costs, (2) health-care costs, (3) health-care costs. No ambivalence here; the message was not only clear but on target. As national health-care expenditures, having passed $900 billion, approach $1 trillion, the cost of care means different things to different people. To some it is the $10,000 or more for one day's hospitalization in intensive care. For others it is represented by the $18.3 million total compensation (salary, bonuses, and stock options) for the chairman of an entrepreneurial multihospital system. The upward slope of physicians' incomes since the enactment of Medicare, rising to seven times the average per capita income, is both a culprit and a consequence.[3]

For some physicians, excessive health-care costs can be found in their premiums for malpractice coverage; "professional liability insurance" can cost over $100,000 a year in selected specialities in some urban areas. For medical students, health-care costs represent indebtedness of as much as $150,000 at graduation. For a number of elderly individuals, out-of-pocket costs of prescription medications for chronic diseases can be measured in thousands of dollars a year, a substantial proportion of their Social Security checks. A United States senator or representative is apt to see the public-sector share of total cost as a trade-off with expenditures for education, housing, social welfare, energy, the environment, the infrastructure, and national security, not to mention as a major contribution to the budget deficit.

Detailed data calculate health-care expenditures in categories such as hospitalization, physician services, pharmaceuticals, and nursing homes. Outcomes and value achieved for the money spent are far more difficult to calculate or document. Health-care costs will be increasingly measured against health-care outcomes. Brian Abel-Smith, a health economist at the London School of Economics, appropriately titled a book *Value for Money in Health*. In health care it is possible to spend more but get less value if value is measured as health status for the population. The iron triangle of access, quality, and cost containment helps us define value. Increasing quality or access adds value, but then so does lowering costs if what we seek is cost-effectiveness. Costs, like access and quality and, for that matter, health itself, are relative.

Prenatal, Neonatal, and Infant Care

The United States ranks twenty-first among members of the United Nations in its rate of infant mortality—the number of newborns out of every 1,000 live births who do not survive to age one.[4] The infant mortality rates in several urban regions would qualify the United States as a third-world country. Infant survival is influenced by more than prenatal care, delivery, and postnatal medical and nursing support. The nutrition of the mother to be, her decision to seek care, and her avoidance of deleterious habits such as drug abuse, cigarette smoking, and consumption of alcohol are just some of the social, cultural, and related variables.

Teenage pregnancy represents a subset of the issues surrounding infant mortality. Consequences can include an end to formal education when the mother drops out of high school, the beginning or perpetuation of a cycle of welfare dependency, and the loss to society of a productive and fully participating citizen. To list teenage pregnancy as a health problem considerably understates the case. Teenage pregnancy is indeed a health problem, but it is also an educational problem, a social-welfare problem, and most importantly a challenge to community institutions. It demonstrates clearly that health care is broader than medical care. Teenage pregnancy goes to the root of our cultural convictions.

Sex education in the schools and the availability of information about contraception and of contraceptive devices challenge religious values and family beliefs. And yet, until recent advances with in vitro fertilization, every pregnancy was the consequence of a sexual encounter. Sex education alone is not the answer to teenage pregnancy any more than abortion is the answer. Motivation and behavior during that hormonal storm called adolescence must be better understood.

To describe and assess the full spectrum of related issues, such as AIDS and other sexually transmitted diseases, requires interdisciplinary perspectives and strategies devised by an array of specialized talent. Health, educational, and social-welfare programs must work in concert to suggest ways to address the health needs of those affected.

Health Care for the Elderly

"Grow old along with me! The best is yet to be," urged Robert Browning, but his confidence would be hard to justify today. Chronic disease and physical disability, not to mention diminished economic capacity, affect many who are in their seventies, eighties, nineties, and more. When Medicare was enacted in 1965 there were 18 million Americans sixty-five and older—less than 10 percent of the population. A quarter-century after its implementation, there are 32 million older Americans, representing 12.6 percent of the population. Moreover, their average life expectancy extends almost another two decades. Sometime between 2025 and 2030, one in five Americans will be sixty-five or older; in fact, one million Americans will be a hundred or older. Labor projections for the year 2030 indicate we will have two gainfully employed workers contributing to the Social Security trust fund for each person eligible for benefits.[5] In 1945, fifty contributors supported each potential beneficiary. If health-care costs were to continue to rise as they have in the last two decades, by 2030 the Medicare program would draw on an economy devoting approximately 50 percent of the gross domestic product to health and medical care. Something has to give.

Most men and women over sixty-five suffer from four or more chronic diseases, such as arthritis, hypertension, diminished vision, and hearing loss. These conditions require health services for maintenance of function and minimization of disability. Total hip arthroplasty (hip replacement) and surgical extraction of cataracts with lens implant are critical among these services. The prescription drugs most widely utilized by the elderly are anti-inflammatory agents, but one popular medication, a nonsteroidal agent, can cost in excess of $1,000 per year. Major benefits are to be found in expenditures for corrective lenses, hearing aids, canes, and walkers. Prevention of home accidents (adequate lighting, crash bars in bathrooms, and amplified phones) and social-support services are highly cost-effective. The elderly gain more benefit in functional capacity from physical therapists, social workers, podiatrists, and nutritionists than they do from many medical specialists.

AIDS

Acquired Immune Deficiency Syndrome challenges the boundaries of health policy across our society. The Centers for Disease Control estimated 115,000 to 170,000 United States residents with AIDS in 1992,[6] and the number is expected to increase by between 139,000 and 205,000 by 1995. During the past five years, new cases have risen from 1,500 per month to more than 4,000. By 1995, the cumulative total of AIDS patients in the United States is expected to range from 400,000 to 550,000.

The tragedy, of course, derives from the disease's universal fatality in two to six years from onset. By the turn of the century, the cumulative death toll in the United States will be between 600,000 and 1.3 million. The human misery cannot be quantified. Adding to the tragedy are estimated direct health-care expenditures of $15 billion by 1995. The total cost for hospitalization and treatment of an AIDS patient can exceed $100,000, and a disproportionate number of victims are poor—and therefore uninsured. Moreover, when a person with AIDS loses a job, he or she loses insurance as well; people who have AIDS or are HIV-positive cannot get insurance.

Sir William Osler, revered as the most distinguished clinician of the early twentieth century, observed, "To know syphilis is to know medicine."[7] The all-pervasiveness of that disease's symptoms, signs, and pathophysiology, which challenged the medical knowledge of his time, supported the observation. In the 1990s, to know AIDS is to know public health, as well as medicine, and to appreciate the diverse dimensions of health policy—the organization, financing, and delivery of health services—in addition to the immunology, epidemiology, and pharmacology of AIDS. The American health-care enterprise is tested as never before.

Abortion

Pro-choice and pro-life demonstrators take to the streets to rally public opinion to their causes. Increasingly, when the two factions meet at an abortion clinic, a nonviolent demonstration becomes a highly charged conflict in which each side claims a truth that the other considers fanaticism. Law-enforcement officials are caught in the middle trying to restore calm and, one would hope, civil discourse. In the midst of this, scientists conclude that they are unable to determine when life begins. In the final decade of the twentieth century, abortion could surpass virtually all other issues in its political significance and its implications for health-care reform.

It too, however, may be affected by societal and technoscientific forces outside the current debate. The development of RU-486, the so-called morning-after pill, could make the arguments moot, or at least move them to the departments of philosophy or the divinity schools of universities. Although the drug, developed in France, is not yet available in the United States, testing is now on the agenda. Its availability could create a fine line between taking the oral contraceptive pill before or the abortion pill after. What many consider a health issue and what others argue is a moral one may at last become a private matter between a woman and her physician. Biomedical technology can and often does provoke cultural, economic, and political changes in society. For the moment, though, the issue of abortion will necessarily figure in debates on health-care reform.

Substance Abuse

Substance abuse, even more than teenage pregnancy, is a challenge to health services, educational programs, and social-welfare initiatives; it is a challenge as well, of course, to the criminal-justice system. There is conflict between health-care agencies and law-enforcement agencies on correct approaches, although one urban mayor, Kurt L. Schmoke of Baltimore, has advocated learning from the lessons of Prohibition: focus on public-health measures rather than on criminal justice.[8] When the dealers and users are of school age, the issues become even more complex.

Far from being restricted to problems like crack addiction, substance abuse is also used as a damning term for cigarette smoking. In 1964 the surgeon general, Luther L. Terry, warned of the health hazards. Two decades later another surgeon general, C. Everett Koop, called for a smoke-free society after the year 2000.[9] There is clear evidence of nicotine addiction and the lethal carcinogenic properties of tobacco smoke. Yet the economic factors for the tobacco farmer, not to mention the profits for manufacturers and distributors, are formidable.

American society has clearly given the individual the freedom to assume risk in the pursuit of pleasure. On the other hand, millions of nonsmokers would agree with Poor Richard's adage that "your liberty ends where my nose begins." A smoke-free environment on commercial airline flights and in workplaces, restaurants, and other public spaces is evidence of the concern over passive smoking. Moreover, cigarettes appear to be every legislator's favorite tax vehicle.

Wine, unlike cigarettes, has a significant ritualistic use in many religions, and moderate consumption of wine with meals has been advocated by nutritional authorities as possibly contributing not only to a sense of well-being but to one's health. The impact of imprudent consumption, however, is widely known; alcoholism is a significant health problem.

Surplus of Physicians and Shortage of Nurses

Public policy has concerned itself for some three decades now with the relative numbers of physicians and nurses (currently about 650,000 and 2.3 million).[10] Contributing to the problem of too many physicians and too few nurses is the widespread perception in both professions that the tasks and responsibilities of each are not readily transferable, especially as the extraordinary specialization within medicine has increasingly been mirrored within nursing. It can no longer be said that a physician is a physician is a physician or a nurse is a nurse is a nurse: these once generic roles have yielded to specialties and subspecialties. A radiologist cannot be expected to provide the services of a family physician; nor can an intensive-care-unit nurse substitute for a nurse midwife.

Two-thirds of the physicians in the United States—far more, proportionately, than in Canada or the United Kingdom—are specialists, representing a variety of skills and technological preferences to which the patient has virtually random access. Instead of a family physician, a typical family can have an obstetrician and gynecologist for the mother, a pediatrician for the young children, a sports-medicine specialist for the adolescents, an internist or perhaps cardiologist for the father, a gerontologist or nurse practitioner for the grandparents, and a family therapist to tie everything together.

In 1980, the Graduate Medical Education National Advisory Commission (GMENAC), examining the nation's needs for physicians, predicted a surplus of 145,000 by the year 2000. The commission members foresaw, however, a shortage of pediatricians, physical-medicine and rehabilitation physicians, and some other specialists.[11] In nursing, conversely, one could find a surplus of certain specialities within an overall shortage.

Some solutions to the perceived nursing shortage have been proposed recently by Linda H. Aiken and Connie Flynt Mullinex, whose authoritative study suggests expansion of nursing-school enrollments, recruitment of inactive nurses, and greater utilization of part-time nurses and nurses trained abroad. But the crux of the problem is the necessity to restructure hospitals, the principal employers of professional nurses, so as to use nursing expertise as effectively as possible.[12]

There is no simple formula for meeting a society's requirements for physicians and nurses. Considerations of desirable population ratios, acceptable expenditures, and minimum standards will each yield different target figures. Finally, though, the real concern ought to be the availability and quality of care, the character of skills, concerns, and services rather than numbers. How physicians and nurses are utilized in various delivery systems will do much to determine the ways that the society addresses the need to balance access, quality, and cost.

Medical Tort Reform

Law and medicine derive from disparate cultures with differing definitions of truth. To the physician, truth is arrived at when a disease fulfills Koch's postulates for confirming the etiologic agent or when a random-control trial yields a P value of less than .001, meaning the observed event would occur by chance alone only once in a thousand occurrences. For the lawyer, truth is achieved when proper judicial procedure monitors adversarial counsel, the rules of evidence prevail, and a jury of one's peers renders a verdict.

No subject can enrage a practicing physician as rapidly as malpractice, or professional liability, can. Most physicians agree with the principle that they are accountable to the local standards of practice, and they seek to care for their patients accordingly. Responsible lawyers endorse this commitment. Here the agreement ends. Physicians feel under attack by ungrateful patients and charlatan attorneys and are convinced that contingency fees—legal fees calculated as a percentage of the judgment—invite open season on physicians by 850,000 lawyers, many of whom are looking for work. Moreover, physicians are convinced that society's expectations for perfection and guaranteed outcomes do not take into account such occurrences as congenital malformations, over which physicians have no control. Lawyers, of course, believe that every individual has a right to his or her day in court.

For society at large, a major concern is the cost of malpractice litigation. Awards and lawyers' fees are the direct costs. Expenditures for services aimed at documenting and justifying clinical services come under the rubric "defensive medicine." Hence the ankle X ray even when the physician in the emergency room is convinced there's only a sprain, or the gastroscopy with a flexible fiberoptiscope to confirm the symptoms of a peptic ulcer—a couple of decades ago, a patient would have had a diagnostic trial of antacids.

The medical profession is a science, an art, and a business. The resolution of malpractice suits by settlement or verdict most directly influences the business of medicine; but their causes are more usually related to the art, while the court arguments focus on the science.

Some form of arbitration, with an agreed-on set of criteria, standards, and procedures, offers hope for a balance between the physician's clinical judgment and the lawyer's advocacy of the patient's right to redress.

Disease Prevention and Self-Health Promotion

Healthy behavior is an arena in which we have much control over our destinies, with or without the intervention of health professionals. Perhaps the most critical choice is the selection of one's parents: heredity, or more precisely our underlying genetic makeup, is a major template of our health status. Short of genetic engineering in some future era, our genetic legacy reflects a random destiny. Nevertheless, certain imperatives for healthy living have been identified: eat three low-fat meals, particularly breakfast, daily and avoid snacks; sleep seven to eight hours each night; exercise regularly; drink alcohol only in moderation; do not smoke cigarettes; wear a seat belt when driving, or riding in, a motor vehicle.[13]

The area of mental health is also a major concern, and coverage of pertinent services is an important focus of debate over health-care reform. It has been some time since mental-health services were strictly the domain of psychiatrists and psychopharmacologists; provision of such services is widely defused through clinical psychologists, psychiatric social workers, clergy with training in counseling, personal support groups, and many others.

The lay referral system identified over thirty years ago is now becoming the lay therapeutic system.[14] Thus many activities directed at promoting health and preventing disease are almost totally outside the health-care enterprise. As these phenomena become more diffuse and widespread, one can expect the lay referral system to shape the decisions of more and more people, many of whom may seek counsel and support elsewhere than in doctors' offices and in clinics.

Right to Die

Approximately 30 percent of the total expenditures for hospitalization under Medicare occur within the last year of patients' lives.[15]

Daniel Callahan, director of the Hastings Institute; Richard D. Lamm, former governor of Colorado; and John Silber, president of Boston University, among others, consider this resource expenditure disproportionate, inappropriate, and socially irresponsible. A highly charged issue, the problem of cost often immediately raises questions about euthanasia. There are far easier ways to begin the discussion.

The Wissahickon Hospice has cared for more than 3,000 terminally ill people living in the northwest section of Philadelphia and in the adjacent county. Approximately 85 percent of these patients have died of cancer. Self-referred or referred by physicians, nurses, and social workers, patients choose to receive terminal care at home rather than to undergo technological heroics. They seek control of pain and the opportunity to live out their lives in familiar and comfortable surroundings. The Wissahickon Hospice staff finds that the patients and their families are often more willing to accept the finite dimensions of life than are their medical caregivers.

Euthanasia (from the Greek, meaning "easy death") became a best-selling topic in 1991 when Derek Humphry, founder of the Hemlock Society, published *Final Exit*, a slim handbook on how to end one's life. The difficulty and the agony of the decision to assist the death of a terminally ill patient were poignantly described by a physician, Timothy Quill, in the *New England Journal of Medicine*. And another doctor, Jack Kevorkian, has made a crusade of pursuing the issue of assisted suicide into the courts.[16]

Passive action to let life run its course is far different from active intervention to hasten death. Moreover, the individual patient's desire to avoid technology is different from a professional's making the decision to pull the plug. Living wills and advanced directives are increasingly being adopted as vehicles for individuals to make known to health professionals their desire not to receive specific treatments that may prolong life or the dying process. The instructions must be communicated to and accepted by family members before they can be fully effective.

The ethical debate does not occur only at the end of life. Sustaining the life of a premature infant can be even more expensive and psychologically draining and can have grave long-term consequences. Thirty years ago, it took heroic measures to save an infant weighing 2,500 grams (the average birth weight today is 3,500 grams). Soon we were down to 2,000, then 1,500, and then 1,000 grams. Now neonates weighing 750 grams or less have a fighting chance, though against formidable odds and at great cost. Where, if at all, will we draw the line? In some European countries very low-birth-weight infants might not be treated, but in the United States they represent a challenge. Medical technology and ethics are joined in resource allocation.

When, in 1964, Lyndon Johnson appointed the President's Commission on Heart Disease, Cancer, and Stroke, to be chaired by the distinguished heart surgeon Michael DeBakey, he noted that these three diseases accounted for two-thirds of American deaths but forecast that their conquest would contribute to an average life expectancy of a hundred years in the twenty-first century.

After nine months of study, the commission brought forth almost three dozen recommendations that addressed research, training, planning, public-health programs, and regionalized systems emanating from academic health centers.[17] Today heart disease, cancer, and stroke remain the leading causes of death, but individuals are living longer and more adaptive lives with these diseases. We all die of something, though, and even if one leading cause of death is eliminated, another merely takes its place. After all, when the FBI catches one of its ten most-wanted criminals, someone else is added to the list.

For much of the history of health affairs in American society the focus has been on increasing life expectancy—that is, the years of life. Health-care reform must address the quality of life for those years. The next chapter analyzes the character of the quest.

Chapter 3
An Infinite Quest

*A healthy individual can be defined
as someone who has been inadequately
studied.*

Health is an elusive concept, difficult to define and virtually
impossible to measure. Diagnostic skills are aimed primarily at finding
or quantifying the indicators of dis-ease, or the lack of comfort. How
can one identify, describe, and measure health with sufficient precision to know when it has been achieved? Moreover, is health to be
determined objectively, subjectively, or both ways? Is health an end in
itself or a means to achievement?

In an introductory graduate course on health-care management for
students from a variety of backgrounds, I ask two of them to volunteer
for an informal survey. A business student evaluates the health status
of his colleague. His questions invariably focus on function, performance in class, feelings of well-being and optimism, or anticipated
activities. There are no questions about disease or medical status. I ask
another student, a physician, to conduct an interview. Questions focus
on chief complaints (why else would anyone consult a physician?) and
proceed through present illness, personal history, family history, and
review of symptoms.

The first interview illustrates the consumer's perspective on health; the second demonstrates the physician's relentless search for disease. If my physician student had been permitted a physical examination of her colleague and had found nothing wrong, she could turn to dozens of laboratory, diagnostic, and imaging technologies. If all else failed, a probe of the subject's psyche would likely yield some abnormality, as it would with anyone else. Physicians are trained to document the anatomy, biochemistry, and pathology of the imperfections borne by each of us.

Medicine seeks to eliminate the negative while the nursing model seeks to emphasize the positive in the patients' capacity to function. To a nurse, each patient represents the challenge to increase performance. To a physician, a healthy individual is someone who has been inadequately studied.

Life-expectancy, mortality, and morbidity rates provide surrogate measures of health status. Should we try to measure health by performance on a treadmill or by approximation of ideal weight? What about miles jogged, laps swum, oat bran consumed, consecutive days without a cigarette, or moderation in the consumption of alcohol? The designated driver may someday rank alongside polio vaccine as a public-health triumph. These are all means to an end: good health.

The World Health Organization (WHO) defines health as "a state of complete physical, mental, and social well-being and not merely the absence of disease or infirmity."[1] The health agency that speaks for all nations recognizes that considerations of quality of life are appropriate to a philosophy of health. Its definition of health transcends the correction of deficiencies and moves toward the holistic pursuit of harmony in life. René Dubos, a distinguished biological scientist at Rockefeller University, countered the WHO definition of health, however, by noting that "in reality, complete freedom from disease and from struggle is almost incompatible with the process of living."[2]

Dubos discusses the impact on health of technological achievements and social behavior. Scientific and social advances cut two ways. Developments in agricultural technology and a rising standard of living afford most Americans freedom from nutritional deficiencies and contribute to increased life expectancy. At the same time, abundance has encouraged new health problems: fatty degeneration of blood vessels and obesity. Having mastered infectious diseases that formerly took the lives of millions, mainly infants and children, science now must face the chronic and degenerative disorders—cardiovascular disease, cancer, lung disease, and arthritis. In some respects, thus, we have substituted the problems of morbidity for those of mortality. For example, diabetes, a fatal disease during the first decades of the twentieth century, can now be managed as a variation of the metabolic process. The diabetic patient, though, has an increased risk of loss of vision, stroke, and other complications from prolonged diabetes.

Lacking the capacity to identify and measure the positive dimensions of health, we concentrate on the curtailment and elimination of illness, while recognizing that an individual can be diseased without being ill and ill without being diseased. A comprehensive approach to healing, alleviating, or palliating ailments requires an understanding of the human as a social animal with both a soma and a psyche. At present, the biological dimensions of ill health are better understood than the behavioral and functional aspects are.

A hierarchy of health strategies begins with efforts to reduce mortality, particularly in the early decades, and proceeds to reducing serious morbidity, detecting and reducing minor morbidity, and finally enhancing positive health. These emphases also overlap. When society shifts its emphasis from the goal of reducing mortality toward that of promoting positive health, the measurement of progress becomes more difficult. Likewise, although serious morbidity can also usually be accurately diagnosed, it may go undetected for years. Measurement of minor morbidity presents formidable problems, yet for the children, adolescents, and young and middle-aged adults of our society, its measurement becomes critical to ascertaining relative success in attaining health goals.

For the present, the measures of a population's improved health status are an increase in life expectancy, reduction in age-specific mortality rates, and prevention of epidemics and outbreaks of infectious diseases like polio, measles, tuberculosis, and AIDS. Other valid measures are the early detection and cure of diseases with potentially serious morbidity—for example, cancer of the cervix, rheumatic fever, and hypertension—and a decrease in days lost to the labor force because of disability.

A report put out by the U.S. Public Health Service succinctly analyzes what is meant by health status. It defines health as "the effective functioning of an individual in a role appropriate to his age and sex."[3] Health status has been most effectively measured in the young in terms of growth and development, immunizations, and the acquisition of social skills. As the population ages, efforts to measure health status for senior citizens focus on activities of daily living.

What are our desired outcomes? Do we want increased longevity, decreased age-specific mortality, decreased age- and sex-specific morbidity, decreased morbidity from selected diseases, increased quality of life, or the improved productivity that will return the nation to economic competitiveness? Although health cannot be defined within the present limits of scientific knowledge, reduction in the frequency and duration of illness stands as a temporary and determinable goal. It also, however, represents a formidable undertaking.

The Dichotomy of Health Care

One of the most valuable reference guides in medicine is the *Physicians' Desk Reference*, or *PDR*. The 1994 edition, 2,669 pages long, lists and describes approximately 3,000 pharmaceutical agents. The International Classification of Disease (ICD.9.CM) lists thousands of diagnoses and surgical procedures. The range, diversity, and complexity of health services are extraordinary. These services—or, more narrowly, medical care—can be viewed across a continuum from the general and frequent to the complex and rare (table 2). The challenge of health-care reform is to address the entire spectrum.

Physician Factors. The polarization of tertiary care and primary care dramatically affects the work of the physician. The tertiary specialist works predominantly in the hospital with inpatients and within the controls of an institutional setting; the primary-care physician works predominantly in an office, where the social expectations resemble those found in the home and the community. Tertiary care tends to be hierarchical; the ministrations of the primary-care physician usually involve more of a factor of collegiality. Medical education tends to value the characteristics of tertiary care and to undervalue those of primary care.

Table 2
The Dichotomy of Health Care

Primary Care	Tertiary Care
Physician Factors	
Generalist	Specialist
Office/ambulatory	Hospital/inpatient
Home/community	Institutional setting
Matrix organization	Hierarchical orientation
Diagnostic Factors	
10–20% of diagnoses	80–90% of diagnoses
75% of morbidity experience	25% of medical need
Few therapeutic regimens	Extensive treatment protocols
Patient histories	Diagnostic studies
Therapeutic Factors	
Health care	Medical cure
Cognitive	Technique dependent
Symptomatic/placebo	Specific therapies
Minor illness	Serious morbidity
Patient Factors	
Population at risk	Individual need
Continuity	Episodic
Comprehensive	Categorical
Gatekeeper	Referral
Physician: patient (collaborative)	Physician (dominant): patient (submissive)

Diagnostic Factors. It has been estimated that primary care accounts for 10 to 20 percent of all diagnoses and tertiary care for 80 to 90 percent. The specialist's diagnoses account, though, for only about 25 percent of medical need; the few diagnoses of concern to the primary-care physician constitute 75 percent of the morbidity experience in the population. There are, in other words, a few people with complex problems and a lot of people with common problems. Specialists require extensive treatment protocols and diagnostic studies;

primary-care physicians rely more on patient histories and laboratory or minor diagnostic inquires.

Therapeutic Factors. What do the two types of physicians do? The tertiary specialist focuses on medical cure while the primary-care physician takes a functional approach addressed to health care. The specialist works with techniques; the primary-care physician depends more on cognitive skills. Specialists tend to be more attuned to discrete therapies while primary-care physicians more frequently use symptomatic strategies and wait for the organism to respond and overcome the current onslaught. The specialist's therapies are more concerned with serious morbidity, the generalist's with minor illness.

Patient Factors. The need addressed in tertiary care is clearly individual. Primary care is important in the context of the population, in responding, for example, to infectious disease. The concerns of the patient in tertiary care are predominantly episodic and categorical in contrast to the comprehensive and continuous concerns expressed in a primary-care setting. Patients are referred for tertiary care but are more likely to select their primary-care physicians. From the patient's point of view, the relationship with the physician is all-important. In tertiary care, the physician is dominant and the patient submissive; in primary care there is more of a collaborative relationship. An educated patient with a chronic disease is likely to know as much about the disease as the physician does, if not more, and is clearly part of the therapeutic team. Physicians don't really manage diabetes, for example; they educate the patient to help manage his or her condition.

The Demographic Dimension

The Bureau of the Census projects the population of the United States hour by hour. It assumes one birth every 8 seconds, one death every 15, one person immigrating every 32, and one emigrating every 198, for a net gain of one person every 10 seconds. As of 1 January 1994, the figure stood at 259,349,126.[4] That is the first and basic measurement of what medicine terms the population at risk and business calls market niches. In addition to the total census,

status is primarily, but not exclusively, dependent on three intersecting societal institutions: medical care, education, and social welfare. To emphasize these is not, however, to diminish the importance of nutrition, housing, recreation, security, or the environment.

Where the medical model is predominantly disease-oriented and directed toward finding causes, the welfare model emphasizes the functional capacity and economic viability of the individual. Similarly, educational perspectives are concerned with individual potential and accomplishment. The medical model has been very successful in attacking some illnesses, but the other perspectives have been of major importance as well. Where the societal institutions intersect, the achievement of health status becomes an interdisciplinary collaboration. That collaboration is particularly relevant when we ask how society will cope with the problems of AIDS, teenage pregnancy, substance abuse, motor-vehicle accidents, and aging. All three spheres of societal activity become imperative.

The Nation's Health

Fundamental to determining the health status of the population of the United States have been the annual National Health Surveys mandated by the National Health Survey Act of 1956. A survey of 737,000 urban households conducted in 1935–36 had provided a baseline report updated during and after World War II by government and voluntary agencies. The current reports, the "rainbow series" (so called because of their color-coded covers) issued by the National Center for Health Statistics, present the results of household interviews, physical examinations of stratified random samples of the population, specified disease screening, and hospital discharge surveys. They provide ongoing descriptions of the collective health status of 260 million people, documentation of the population's utilization of health services, and records of its payments for those services.[5]

The task at hand is to establish specific goals against which achievements can be measured. The surgeon general's 1979 *Report on Health Promotion and Disease Prevention* advanced five goals, and the Year 2000 Health Objectives Planning Act of 1990 provides legislative support for the development of an explicit prevention program based on those goals.[6] A set of eighteen health-status indicators was developed to assist communities in assessing general health: infant mortality by race and ethnicity; age-adjusted death rates (per 100,000) from motor-vehicle accidents, work-related injuries, suicide, lung cancer, breast cancer, cardiovascular disease, homicide, and all other causes; reported incidence (per 100,000) of AIDS, measles, tuberculosis, and primary and secondary syphilis; the prevalence of such risk factors as low birth weight (less than 2,500 grams), birth to adolescents (ten to seventeen years), no prenatal care in the first trimester, and childhood poverty; and the portion of the population living in counties failing to meet Environmental Protection Agency air-quality standards.[7] These indicators can document change over time.

Like the Year 2000 Health Objectives, they are characteristic of the society's reliance on measurement and quantification. Health, however, is more than numbers. The World Health Organization's definition of health, for example, is hardly a numerical algorithm. Moreover, health values are subjective and derive from spiritual and philosophic conviction; Americans are accustomed to freedom of choice in such values. The implications of these values for care are considered in the next chapter.

Chapter 4
A Cultural Affair

Health care transcends the
biomedical sciences.

Culture, that all-pervasive force, shapes everything we do. Its influence on the delivery of health care can perhaps most readily be seen if one compares the systems in three societies that share a common biomedical literature—the United Kingdom, Canada, and the United States. Despite all the forces tending to homogenize the three cultures, the organization and financing of their health services remain distinct. For many health reformers in the 1990s the Canadian system has replaced that of the United Kingdom as a model for the United States, but both systems demonstrate the role of the cultures in which they are embedded and suggest implications for reform of the American method of health-care delivery.

The British National Health Service

At 260 million, the population of the United States is more than four times that of the United Kingdom. The density of population in the United States, sixty-six persons per square mile, is, however, approximately one-tenth that in the United Kingdom. Ten states have larger land areas than the entire United Kingdom, whose population would fit rather snugly into Oregon. Whereas one can travel from London to Edinburgh in approximately five hours by high-speed train, the same amount of time would not get one from Washington, D.C., to Honolulu in a DC-10.

The National Health Act had its genesis in World War II. The hardship suffered by the British people resulted in a determination to enact ameliorative social programs. The concept of the welfare state for the United Kingdom was developed by William Henry Beveridge, director of the London School of Economics. Unfortunately, he assumed that once all the neglected illnesses had been treated, the demand for health services would decline.

The act called for the minister of health "to promote the establishment in Great Britain of a comprehensive health service." Health care was nationalized, as were many industries. The organization launched in 1948, the National Health Service, functioned with only minor revisions for a quarter-century. Three units were directly responsible to the Department of Health and Social Security for providing comprehensive health care: a general-practitioner service, a hospital and consultant service, and a community health service.

In organizing the general-practitioner service, the National Health Service drew on a precedent established in 1911 under Prime Minister David Lloyd George in which workers were covered for physicians' services by a capitation payment.[1] General practitioners characteristically functioned in solo practices, often in offices, or "surgeries," in their homes.

All hospitals were nationalized. They were suffering from a severe shortage of capital, having had virtually no infusion of financial resources during the Depression or World War II. Traditionally, in the United Kingdom, specialists occupied staff positions in hospitals. In a compromise between the government and the medical societies, consultants were permitted to maintain part-time private practices. Private patients could pay for beds in the teaching hospitals where the specialists who admitted them served on contract.

Local health authorities—or public-health services, as Americans know them—incorporate maternal and child health care, health visitors in the home, community nursing and midwifery, school programs, and other preventive and follow-up services.

A study undertaken in 1970 to evaluate organizational initiatives for improving the provision of health services acknowledged at the outset that a population of 55 million was too large for significant program planning and development.[2] A reorganization of the National Health Service began in 1974 and represented management restructuring on an unprecedented scale. A total of 227 districts were organized to plan and implement the medical and health services for populations of approximately 250,000. In each district, an administrator, a nurse, a financial officer, and a community physician provided consensus management. Community health councils were established to evaluate the performance of hospitals and services. Joint consultative committees provided coordination between local governments and eighty-eight area health authorities, each representing approximately three districts. They reported to fifteen regional health authorities, which focused on allocation of resources and strategic planning. Medical advisory committees at the district, area, and regional levels completed the organizational schema.

It didn't take long for the Department of Health and Social Security to find the 1974 plan inordinately cumbersome. There appeared to be too many layers. In 1981 another reorganization attempted to streamline the National Health Service by essentially merging the district management teams with the area health authorities to create district health authorities. The hierarchical management structure controlling resource allocation remained.

The 1980s saw a series of white papers, inquiries, and reports addressed to strategies for more effective management and budgeting.[3] Drawing on the American experience, many discussed health maintenance organizations and regional markets. The most important recommendation was that funding ought to follow the patient rather than the provider. The district health authorities became responsible for purchasing services. Instead of automatically receiving resources allocated by the Department of Health, hospitals and their consultant staffs had to earn their budgets by attracting patients either directly or through referral by general practitioners. Although today the single payer is still the Exchequer, organizational and funding flexibility like that in Canada and the United States is being sought. As one colleague—Clifford Graham, director of the Institute of Health at King's College in London—says, "We are searching for a mid-Atlantic strategy."

Canadian National Health Insurance

The 3,000-mile border shared by the United States and Canada is freely crossed by the technological advances of modern medicine. Moreover, as Canadian national health insurance confronts the reality of resource scarcity, some patients are traveling to the United States for certain high-tech procedures. But the organization, financing, and delivery of health services are society-specific, reflecting several differing national characteristics. Differences of geography and scale are especially important. Canada, with the same area as the United States, has one-tenth its population.

The passage of the British North America Act in 1867 established Canada as a constitutional monarchy and a federated state with a government based on the British parliamentary system, which effectively provides no separation between legislative and executive branches of government. The act did, however, specify a division of powers between the federal and provincial levels of government, and historically the role of the provinces has been strong. Indeed, the combined provincial budgets exceed the budget of the federal government.

The constitution of Canada was returned to full Canadian control by the British Parliament only in 1982. Apart from the continuing British influence, there is that of the French Canadian segment of the population, and there are sizable contingents representing farm and socialist interests. These are some of the diverse influences that affect the national health program.

In 1945 federal subsidies to the provinces for health programs were considered in the Canadian House of Commons, and in 1947 the province of Saskatchewan passed legislation providing for mandatory hospital insurance, the first such coverage in North America, guaranteeing an entire population virtually unlimited care in general hospitals. British Columbia followed in 1949, and Alberta in 1950.

The passage of legislation governing hospital insurance in the three most western provinces, along with a series of federal and provincial conferences, set the stage for the Hospital Insurance and Diagnostic Services Act of 1957. The federal government offered to provide 50 percent funding for the provincial hospital insurance plans, which provided comprehensive inpatient services, universal coverage, equal access for all provincial residents, and portability of benefits from one province to another. By 1961 all provinces and territories had taken advantage of the federal subsidy. The province of Saskatchewan again led the way, by passing legislation providing for insurance covering physicians' fees. The passage of this legislation in 1962 resulted in a physicians' strike in the province.

In 1961 the federal government appointed a Royal Commission on Health Services to "examine the question of unmet needs in Canadian health care." Its report, issued in 1964, recommended federal subsidization of provincially administered medical-care insurance.[4] In 1966 the Medical Care Act was passed, but federal budget constraints delayed implementation until 1968. Also, by June 1968 only British Columbia and Saskatchewan had met the eligibility requirements. The act provided 50 percent federal subsidization of provincial medical insurance plans that met five criteria: universality (coverage of at least 95 percent of the population), comprehensive services, portability, public administration, and reasonable access to insured services. By 1972 all provinces had established qualifying programs.

The Established Programs Financing Act of 1977 changed the open-ended matching formula to a per capita block-grant approach, with annual increases indexed to the overall nominal growth in the gross domestic product. The result was an increased financial burden on the provinces. The fourth major legislative initiative, the Canadian Health Act, passed in 1984, effectively eliminated fees for hospital services and extra billing by physicians. All provinces eliminated extra billings and user charges by March 1987. Once again physicians went on strike, this time in Ontario.

National health insurance in Canada, a decentralized program based on ten provinces, suggests a principle similar to that of Medicaid, with its federal subsidy of health services through the fifty state governments. The disparity among the states as to eligibility, level of coverage, and duration, however, contrasts starkly with the universality, comprehensiveness, portability, and equity of access that are fundamental to the Canadian scheme. Development of the program has spanned four decades, from the passage of the National Health Act in 1948 to the 1957 Hospital Insurance and Diagnostic Services Act, the 1966 Medical Care Act, the 1977 Established Programs Financing Act, and the 1984 Canadian Health Act.[5]

The United States: Pluralism in Search of Excellence

When King George VI gave his assent to the British National Health Act in 1946, he provided the American Medical Association with a straw man against which to rail; when Harry Truman proposed his national health program in 1948, the AMA sought to discredit it by attacking socialized medicine. There were medical-care reformers in the United States in the 1950s, however, who advocated the British National Health Act as a panacea for the ills of health care in America. Today Canada is the panacea. These idealized perceptions tend to ignore both the deficiencies as well as the real strengths of the British and Canadian systems and the extraordinary cultural disparities among the English-speaking peoples.

The United States is an ethnically pluralistic society with diverse subcultures and, as noted by several observers, a disproportionate "underclass." Canada uses government as an instrument to seek common values and devise derivative programs; the United States appears to prefer government as an instrument for promoting special interests. The words inscribed on the Statue of Liberty—"Give me your tired, your poor, your huddled masses yearning to breathe free"—connote a preference for opportunity over equity. Accordingly, the American health-care enterprise seems likely to continue to address the problem of infinite needs and finite resources by pursuing excellence over equity. By contrast, Canada and the United Kingdom have demonstrated the priority of equity through universality of access.

In the spring of 1975, I addressed a meeting of the Kent Medical Association, the British equivalent of a state medical society. The secretary of the British Medical Association introduced me as "a professor of medicine from the colonies," and I responded in kind. "To appreciate the differences between health care in the colonies and the mother country," I said, "you must recognize that you organize your health services the way we in America play football and we organize our health services the way you play rugby." I meant that access to the disciplined structure of general practitioners and specialists in the National Health Service calls to mind the way two football teams line up in formation, awaiting the snap of the ball. Americans' random access to virtually any physician suggests a rugby scrum in which players locked cheek to jowl flail for the ball. While difficult to describe, the American health-care enterprise can be characterized as flexible, innovative, and variable.

For some Americans, health care is a right fulfilled by the public sector. For others, it is an earned or negotiated benefit by virtue of employment. Some are dependent on the commitment of a religious order. More often than not, health care in the United States is a mixture of two or more of the above, though still not the societal right that it is in the United Kingdom and Canada. A completely comparable consensus in American society will be difficult to achieve. After all, Canada and the United Kingdom have something the United States does not—a unity of government in a parliament. But it has something they don't—a thousand registered health lobbyists, figuratively a fourth branch of government. Individually and collectively they have a formidable impact on the health-policy process.

The process begins with the federal government and its tripartite balance of powers among the executive, legislative, and judicial branches (see fig. 4). Each branch has ramifications for health care in different ways: health-care reform originated in the executive branch; but the Congress, in enacting and appropriating, will support some health initiatives over others, and the Supreme Court may have a singular impact by deciding, for example, whether abortion will be a covered benefit. State and local governments act independently and also in concert with the federal government in various arenas. Dominant in health affairs at the state level are public-health laws, Medicaid programs, workers' compensation, and insurance commissions. The states may have an enhanced role in health-care reform.

Corporations and organized labor, while they occasionally act together, are often at odds when it comes to health policy. National health insurance has long been supported by organized labor. Now

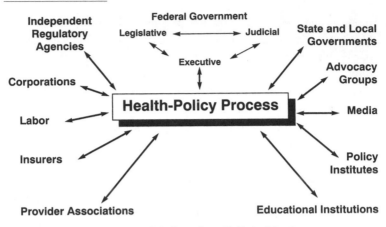

Source: Adapted from National Health Policy Forum, George Washington University

Fig. 4. The Creation of Health Policy

some corporations are looking to national health insurance to standard-ize their share of the burden of health-care coverage. It should be remembered that corporations and labor collaborated during World War II to provide the foothold for third-party coverage of hospital and physician services, primarily through Blue Cross and Blue Shield. Government was the payer. Labor and management each benefited as coverage increased. Insurers, represented independently and collec-tively, and the Blue Cross/Blue Shield Association likewise have a vested interest.

Policy institutes based in Washington and on university campuses have strong research interests and varying degrees of objectivity; they can be found speaking for the left, the center, and the right. Widely known and influential are the Brookings Institution, the RAND Corpo-ration, and the Heritage Foundation. On the same side of the diagram are the media and the advocacy groups, the largest of which is the 34-million-member American Association of Retired Persons.

Provider associations were dominated by the American Medical Association until passage of the Medicare legislation, when they lost out to an alliance of the American Hospital Association, the American Nurses Association, and the AFL-CIO, which supported the legislation. The AMA, with 270,000 physician members, is still very powerful, but physicians are also represented by a number of other associations, such as the American College of Physicians, with 70,000 members. More than fifty physician associations are active in lobbying for programs and influencing policy. A number of physicians are members of several associations. Nurses and other health professionals have a number of associations, as do both voluntary, not-for-profit hospitals and taxpaying, investor-owned ones. Educational institutions are deeply interested in health policy, and some have full-time staffs in Washington to lobby Congress.

Whereas in the 1950s a member of Congress could be expected to consult the family physician or the county medical society on prospective health legislation, no such preemptive position prevails today. Moreover, the representative will seek not only the views of a variety of health professionals but also those of his constituents, who are, after all, patients and consumers. Organized labor, particularly the AFL-CIO, the United Auto Workers, and the teamsters, declare their positions on health issues. When one adds all the voluntary health associations—such as the American Cancer Society and the American Heart Association—as well as the business roundtables; the policy institutes; the advocacy groups; Prudential, Metropolitan Life, CIGNA, Aetna, and other large health insurers; the *Fortune* 500 corporations, which pay a substantial portion of health-care costs; and of course the state and local governments, which participate in Medicaid and carry a significant number of other health responsibilities, one has a health-policy process that reflects the pluralism of the society.

Comparing Systems

Americans treasure diversity and social mobility. British values and expectations tend to be more predictable than those in American society, with its considerable cultural heterogeneity. British notions of royalty, nobility, and class contrast with the ideal of mobility in the United States. Class especially tends to reinforce structure and discipline.

Authority is consulted and respected in the United Kingdom. In our society, freedom of choice is the central priority, and the individual is encouraged to seek out options and select from among them. Authority, while hardly lacking in American society, does not have the same dimension as it does in the United Kingdom. When a British general practitioner sees a patient, reaches a preliminary conclusion, prescribes medication or other measures, and requests the patient to return in ten days, the probability is very high that the patient will comply with the prescribed course and return as instructed. The American patient might well seek a second or third opinion, check with a pharmacist and a neighbor, and never be seen again. The British general practitioner has the use of the most valuable diagnostic tools—time and follow-up observation. The authority of the physician is fundamental in the National Health Service.

So is waiting one's turn. The waiting list for specialist services, mainly elective surgery for patients referred by general practitioners, is a key to the performance of the National Health Service. This mechanism of resource allocation is perceived by most British citizens not as rationing but as the accepted societal norm. "Queuing" for health services works because each person expects that the next person will respect the queue.

A general outline of selected aspects of all three systems illustrates some of the differences that arise from cultural assumptions—and pinpoints, too, some of the similarities.

Type of Practice. Approximately two-thirds of the physicians in the United States are medical specialists. In the United Kingdom, most are in general practice. In Canada, approximately half the physicians are certified as general practitioners or family physicians. The trend, however, is toward increased specialization.

Physician Compensation. The predominant mechanism for paying physicians in the United States is fee for service. In the United Kingdom, specialists receive salaries budgeted by the hospitals where they have consultant appointments; general practitioners receive practice allowances (salary subsidies), capitation payments per enrollee per month (for a total of 60 percent of annual income), and fees for priority services—for example, family planning, cancer screening, and immunization. Although the method of paying physicians in Canada resembles that in the United States, Canadian physicians have a binding fee schedule that each provincial health plan has negotiated with the provincial medical association. Billing beyond the fee schedule is not permitted.

Access to Medical Care. In the United States, one has random access to any generalist, specialist, health maintenance organization (HMO), or preferred provider organization (PPO). A general practitioner in the British National Health Service is responsible for a defined population of patients, usually about 2,300. Access to specialists is by referral. In Canada, access to medical care is universal, comprehensive, and portable to any generalist, specialist, or hospital.

Mode of Practice. Solo practice and partnerships predominate in the United States, with increasing numbers of HMOs, PPOs, and hospital-physician joint ventures. Until recently, most general practitioners in the United Kingdom were in solo practice, but there are more and more small (two- or three-) physician partnerships. Specialists, of course, occupy salaried posts in hospitals. Physicians in Canada participate in group practices to a lesser extent than physicians do in the United States. Participation in independent practice associations (IPAs), PPOs, and HMOs is also not as extensive as in the United States.

Institutional Patterns. In the United States, a majority of short-term general hospitals are voluntary, tax-exempt institutions operated on a not-for-profit basis and accountable to the community through boards of trustees. Approximately 10 percent of such hospitals are in multihospital systems operated for profit and accountable to the investors owning shares. In the United Kingdom the mechanism for distributing resources has been regional, through hospitals owned and run by the government. In Canada, 95 percent of hospitals are not-for-profit or public institutions whose sole source of revenue is the provincial health plan. The remaining 5 percent are facilities for long-term care. Volunteer organizations, municipal and county corporations, provincial authorities, and religious orders are responsible for half of these; the rest are for-profit.

Goals and Objectives. The American health-care system encourages institutional quality so as to provide the best for those who gain access. The strategy in the United Kingdom is one of access, equity, and community orientation. The Canadian strategy falls somewhere between the two other systems.

Source of Health-Care Funds. In the United States, 42 percent of the health-care dollar is from government, 28 percent from third parties, and 30 percent from out of pocket. Despite recent increased privatization of health care in the United Kingdom, almost 90 percent of the health-care pound comes from general revenues and the remainder from voluntary insurance or out of pocket. In Canada, the federal government provides 32 percent and provincial governments 41 percent of health-care expenditures. Private sources represent a quarter, with local governments and workers' compensation providing 2 and 1 percent respectively.

Resource Consumption. The United States spends more than twice as much of its gross domestic product (14 percent) as does the United Kingdom (6.6 percent). Canada, with 10 percent, lies at the midpoint.

Health Status. By current measures of longevity, age-specific mortality, and functional capacity, the health statuses of the United States, United Kingdom, and Canada are virtually identical. This fact begs the real question: to what degree is health status a consequence of medical care? Alternatively, what do other factors contribute?

Eclecticism in health affairs often yields a hybrid vigor. A century ago, for example, Johns Hopkins University combined the model of the German research institutes for students' preclinical studies with the model of the full-time specialists at the London Teaching Hospital for their clinical years. This strategy for medical education at the graduate level was predicated on a foundation of premedical education provided at the undergraduate level by colleges and universities. In 1910 the Hopkins model was endorsed in a landmark study of medical education conducted by Abraham Flexner for the Carnegie Foundation for the Advancement of Education. His report has dominated medical education in the United States for the entire twentieth century.[6]

Canadian medical education has replicated the American model. When McMaster University of Hamilton, Ontario, organized a new medical school in 1965, however, it launched significant innovations in the Flexnerian model. Subsequently several medical schools in the United States have adopted components of the McMaster curriculum.

When the planners in the Office of the Surgeon General of the U.S. Public Health Service developed the proposal for the Hospital Survey and Construction Act of 1946, they drew extensively on the concept of regionalization of hospitals formulated in the United Kingdom by Lord Dawson.[7] The concept proved less transferable, however, than the technology of the CAT scan decades later.

In the 1950s, the idea of a therapeutic community for psychiatric care was developed in the United Kingdom; it became an organizing principle for acute psychiatric services in community hospitals in the United States and helped launch the movement for community mental-health centers in the 1960s. At present, gerontologists in the United States are studying the community strategies for care of the elderly in Edinburgh and Glasgow. One prominent result of cross-cultural borrowing is so-called alternative medicine, incorporating acupuncture from China, relaxation therapy and yoga from India, and holistic strategies from Native Americans. Midwifery is experiencing some growth in our society, while in Germany midwives assist the vast majority of births.

To date, the HMO model for organizing and delivering health services has not appealed significantly in Canada or the United Kingdom. American health-policy analysts are studying the Canadian single-payer system for health-care financing. Perhaps the most dominant feature of the Canadian ethos is the conviction that government is a legitimate, if not the preferred, instrument for the provision of human services. That is a long way from the traditional American idea that the government which governs best is that which governs least.

On the horizon is perhaps the most ambitious cross-cultural experiment in health affairs. Since the 1981 reorganization of the British National Health Service, there has been debate about responding to the consumer and improving efficiency and effectiveness in the organization and delivery of services.[8] Health-care reform in the United Kingdom seems to parallel proposed changes in the United States, with both countries appearing to be searching for a common theory of

Table 3
A Mid-Atlantic Strategy

National Health Service	Health-Care Reform
Exchequer	Global budget
Department of Health	National Health Board
Health authorities	Health alliances
Trust hospitals and fund-holding GPs	Accountable health plans

health economics that juxtaposes large-scale purchasers with restructured providers (see table 3). While sharing common principles, a mid-Atlantic strategy will, however, inevitably reflect the separate cultural contexts in which they are realized.

The British National Health Service is still a top-down system centralized in authority and budget. The United States system is predominantly decentralized and bottom-up; Medicare, as a single payer, is top-down for financing but tries to preserve decentralization of organization and initiative. Both countries are now examining the question of top-down and bottom-up systems in search of cost-effectiveness.

The British global budget is maintained by the chancellor of the Exchequer inasmuch as approximately 90 percent of health-care expenditures come out of the public purse. The global budget in the United States, where approximately 30 percent comes from the federal government and 10 percent from state and local governments, is a different challenge. A balance of market, regulatory, and public-sector budgeting will be required if success in constraining costs is to be realized.

The United Kingdom's Department of Health is led by a cabinet officer and staffed by civil servants; the closest analogy in the United States would be the Department of Health and Human Services. The proposed National Health Board would have some but not total autonomy, much like the Federal Reserve Board or the Federal Trade Commission. Proposed responsibilities include definition of a uniform package of benefits and the establishment of measures to achieve a global budget for health services. In this regard a National Health

Board would have functions similar to those of the Department of Health in the United Kingdom.

In the United Kingdom a governmental enterprise, the National Health Service, is pursuing privatization by developing more autonomous delivery systems in the form of self-selecting trust hospitals and fund-holding general practitioners. Health authorities that controlled hospitals through budgets are now allocating funds to these practitioners, who in turn purchase services for their patients from hospitals. Similarly, health authorities function as health-insurance purchasing cooperatives or regional health alliances in managed competition. The fund-holding GPs and the trust hospitals have the potential for creating the equivalent of the accountable health plans that are envisioned in the United States.

Common economic forces will continue to challenge the health-care systems of both societies, as well as of Canada. All three cultures provide contexts within which those forces will shape health care. Health care, after all, transcends the biomedical sciences; it is a cultural affair.

Chapter 5
Resource Allocation

*No society can provide all
the services its population is able to
utilize.*

Health services are not, and cannot be, free. The source of all health-care financing—like the source of all taxes—is the population. The sources and distribution of funds for health care are ultimately what make up a health-care economic policy. Choices must be made. No matter how euphemistically the idea is expressed, the United States rations health care now and it will ration health care in the future. It is time to abandon the myth that we can afford to do everything we may be capable of doing for every patient. Institutions, communities, and the society must participate in deciding who will benefit.

The Health-Care Dollar

Three-quarters or more of the cost of health care in Australia, Canada, France, Germany, Italy, Japan, Sweden, and the United Kingdom are provided by the revenue raised by taxation or by mandatory contributions. Coincidentally, three-quarters of health-care expenditures in the United States derive from two collective sources, the first compulsory, the second voluntary: taxes and third-party insurance. For the country's economic competitors, three-quarters of health-care costs are covered by the public sector as an entitlement, with government control of resource allocation. For the United States, health care is mainly a mix of Social Security entitlement, public welfare, and a prerogative of employment.

Table 4 shows the percentage of gross domestic product expended for health care in 1991 and the percentage of expenditures provided by the public sector in nine economically advanced countries.[1] Canada and the United States spent the highest percentage of the GDP, 10 percent and 13.2 percent respectively. The other seven countries average 8.1 percent. At 41 percent, the American public sector's contribution was by far the lowest.

The taxes that account for that contribution include federal income tax, state income tax, sales tax, corporate tax, inheritance tax, and, in some instances, real-estate tax; the Medicare trust fund, as mandatory social insurance, functions as a tax too. Typically, third-party coverage is in the form of nontaxable fringe benefits to the employee in lieu of taxable wages. Taxpayers were granted a significant tax deduction for out-of-pocket expenditures (expenses in excess of 3 percent of adjusted gross income) into the 1980s. In theory, taxes, third-party, and out-of-pocket funds can be used to purchase the same services and address all

Table 4
Health-Care Expenditures

Country	Percentage of GDP	Public-Sector Percentage
United Kingdom	6.6	86
Italy	8.3	78
Japan	6.8	73
Germany	8.5	78
Australia	8.6	73
Canada	10.0	76
France	9.1	79
Sweden	8.6	91
United States	13.2	41

population groups. In practice, however, almost 95 percent of payments for hospital services derive from governmental or third-party programs. By contrast, prescriptions for medication are paid predominantly out of pocket. Payments to dentists are proportionately more out of pocket than are payments to physicians.

Distribution mechanisms for health care include fees, capitation, salaries, global budgets, and per-case payment. Most societies are experimenting with different payment mechanisms to control expenditures and achieve cost-effectiveness. Like its partners in the world economy, the United States uses a variety of mechanisms for allocating resources among health-care providers. Standardization exists with Medicare, a nationwide program, but even here there is some variability and choice; Medicaid, as a state program, is less standardized. Third-party payment by 1,500 health-insurance carriers ranges from cash reimbursement for the beneficiary's out-of-pocket expenses to capitation payments to HMOs to cover physicians, nurses, other health professionals, and hospitalization.

The sources of health-care funding—government, third party, or out of pocket—do not necessarily determine the mechanism for distribution of the purchasing power. Table 5 illustrates the flow of funds from the primary sources to the ultimate beneficiaries. The pathways can be enormously varied and difficult to trace. Each third-party payer, corporate or governmental, seeks value in health care for the money expended.

It is most improbable that all segments of the population could enjoy equity of access to health services. Cost containment, after all, must always be weighed against access and quality. Using 14 percent of the gross domestic product, the United States has achieved full access to the highest-quality health care for approximately two-thirds of the population. At this rate, what would it cost to achieve full access for all? Alternatively, how would access and quality be balanced if cost-containment efforts brought expenditures down to 8 or 10 percent of the gross domestic product, comparable to the figures for the nations that are the country's economic competitors?

The haves are not likely to be eager to yield their advantage to the have-nots. Perhaps the first test will come with proposals to apply a means test to Medicare—that is, to tax its dollar value; the elderly

Table 5
Flow of Health-Care Dollars

Sources	Payment	Providers	Services	Consumers
Government	Fee for service	Hospitals	Preventive	Pregnant women
Third party	Capitation	Ambulatory clinics	Ambulatory	Children and youth
Out of pocket	Salary	Specialty centers	Inpatient care	Workforce
Combination	Contracts	Nursing homes	Long-term care	Elderly
	Reimbursement	Physicians	Primary	Occupational groups
	Prospective payment	Nurse practitioners	Secondary	Disabled
	Relative-value scales	Dentists	Tertiary	Disadvantaged
	Global budgets	Pharmacists	Rehabilitation	
		Physical therapists	Hospice	
		Social workers		
		Technologists		
		Optometrists		
		Podiatrists		

enjoy national health insurance while 40 million people, mostly young and unemployed, have none. The achievement of universal access for 260 million Americans will require diverse institutional and community initiatives for resource allocation.

Health services can include everything from acute lifesaving to supportive long-term care, from primary care to the latest technological procedures. Not all can be paid for fully without draconian regulation to contain costs. Mechanisms that allocate scarce resources among health services and population groups must allow existing patterns of care to evolve into new delivery systems.

Provider organizations have historically been dominated by physicians and hospitals, often working at cross-purposes. Provider organizations must clarify responsibilities and accountability for services and population groups. Otherwise, inefficiency threatens to overwhelm the enterprise. Moreover, financing must become the means to an end. Multiple mechanisms for financing health services must not obscure the aim of health services: care of people in need.

The Economics of Medicine

Health care in the United States, approaching $1 trillion in annual expenditures, is clearly big business. It is tempting, therefore, to formulate recommendations for reform exclusively in economic terms. But although medicine and economics have much in common conceptually, they are almost antithetical in practice. Physicians are consulted by patients for diagnoses and appropriate therapies. Economists, by contrast, encourage us to declare our goals and then offer to explain the probable consequences of the alternative strategies we might select. Economists are analysts rather than therapists. Moreover, economic prescriptions seldom if ever can be as precise or as free of side effects as many medical therapies are.

Markets are the lifeblood of economics. The two main players—households and firms—are in dynamic equilibrium. Households make demands, and firms supply. Firms provide goods and services in exchange for money; households obtain money in exchange for labor and capital. In health care, the households may be seen as patients and the firms as physicians and hospitals. The equilibrium of supply and demand is guided in theory by the "invisible hand of the market," and economists explain the consequences of our choices. Our choices in health care are more likely to be driven by values or moral sentiment than by economic rationality.[2]

Markets can be assessed in terms of the following principles of perfect competition: a large number of suppliers and purchasers, no single firm controlling price, free entry and exit of suppliers and purchasers, free substitution of products and services, and perfect information accessible to all suppliers and purchasers.[3] Unfortunately, these principles have only limited applicability to health-care markets. It is true that there are many suppliers and purchasers—thousands of hospitals, hundreds of thousands of physicians, more than 2 million nurses, and 260 million potential consumers—and even with recent mergers and acquisitions an ample number of players remain. The other market criteria are more problematic. "No single firm controlling price" is a difficult economic principle to require in health-care markets. The disproportionate influence of just a few hospitals in many communities often depresses nurses' salaries. The dominance of Blue Cross or Blue Shield in some regions yields advantages of discount pricing that are not available to all. This level of market domination in health-care financing would be considered monopolistic in other industries.

"Free entry and exit of suppliers and purchasers" does not exist in health care. Physicians cannot enter practice without being accredited, licensed, and certified; in most specialities, they have to have hospital privileges. Some economists advocate moving toward perfect competition in health care by abolishing licensure. Anyone who wished could practice medicine or dentistry, operate a hospital, or open a nursing home without permission of a governmental licensing body, professional accreditation, or certification. Market forces would prevail, and caveat emptor would guide quality and value.

"Free substitution of products and services" is a problem for an intimate human service dependent on a relationship of trust. Patients tend to allow substitution of technicians but not of a doctor or nurse practitioner.

"Perfect information accessible to all suppliers and purchasers" is far from having been realized in health care. Hospital morbidity data, cost and income statistics, institutional advertising, newspaper science sections, and pharmaceutical promotions in national magazines may disseminate information, but consumers remain largely outside medicine's dialogue.

Perhaps the contrast between markets and health care is best illustrated by the interaction between the party of the first part (households) and the party of the second part (firms). Health care adds the insurer as the party of the third part and the employer as the party of the fourth part. The dynamic equilibrium between household and suppliers becomes a four-part equation that lacks the tension and accountability between the two parties that characterize economic markets.

In health care, the patient (party of the first part) consults the physician (party of the second part), who is paid by Blue Shield (party of the third part), which sells a contract to the employer (party of the fourth part), who provides fringe benefits in lieu of wages to the employee (party of the first part). What goes around comes around, but where is the market equilibrium?

What happens in health care resembles a scene from *Alice in Wonderland*. One need only imagine the physician providing services in the local supermarket rather than in a hospital. The physician meets her patient there, selects the largest shopping cart, and proceeds to make all the purchasing decisions on behalf of the patient, who compliantly follows, pushing the cart. The physician, as the patient's advocate, selects only the finest-quality items and spares no expense. When they reach the checkout counter with the basket overflowing, the physician smiles compassionately, says, "I'll see you next week," then turns and calls out, "Next patient."

The checkout clerk tallies the items and sends the bill to Blue Shield, which sells a contract to Chrysler to cover the physician-patient interaction. Next we hear the CEO at Chrysler complaining that he can't compete with Honda, Toyota, and Hyundai with one hand tied behind his back by exorbitant health-care costs. The patient, of course, doesn't see the problem. He has received abundant high-quality health services without any out-of-pocket costs or even an awareness of the expenditure. To complete the story, the patient happily drives home in his foreign car, which he selected over a American-made product because it cost less.

Cost-Containment Strategies of Managed Care

Efforts to reintroduce discipline in the interaction of the patient and the provider take many forms. Financing of health care has evolved into a maze of inconsistencies, exceptions, adaptations, and almost incomprehensible regulations. Six principal strategies of cost containment seek to bring supply and demand into equilibrium.

PRIOR AUTHORIZATION

Admission to a hospital creates what economists call "moral hazard." The patient is surrounded by technology paid for by a third party. Since a physician makes the decision to admit a patient and determines the procedures and therapies, utilization of services and length of stay are secondary. Prior authorization of admission by insurers was an early initiative designed to contain costs.

SECOND OPINION

Much clinical decision making is a judgment call, and fee-for-service payment gives the physician an incentive to provide diagnostic tests and therapeutic services. Dr. Eugene McCarthy of Cornell–New York Hospital advocated in the early 1970s that recommendations for elective surgical procedures be confirmed by a second physician prior to hospitalization of the patient.[4]

UTILIZATION REVIEW

This is the most extensively implemented approach to cost monitoring. Virtually all community hospitals have utilization-review and quality-assurance committees, which are required for accreditation by the Joint Commission on Accreditation of Healthcare Organizations. With the advent of personal computers, every institution can now collect and analyze statistical data on physician and hospital performance. The challenge, of course, is to identify the criteria most relevant to institutional goals.

DIAGNOSTIC-RELATED GROUPS

Utilization-review research led to the development of diagnostic-related groups, or DRGs. In the mid-1960s, average length of stay, per diem costs, and costs of hospitalization were analyzed by diagnosis at Connecticut's thirty-five general hospitals. The hospital census yielded almost 400 categories, or diagnostic-related groups, that could be used to calculate average costs to be paid to all hospitals per case.[5] Having failed to control health-care costs after some fifteen years of trying, Congress proposed a paradigm shift from retrospective cost-based reimbursement to prospective case-based pricing. The shift moved the frame of reference from the past to the future, bypassing the present. Resource consumption measured by bed days or by number of X rays no longer determined reimbursement; payment reflected a hospital's case mix.

RESOURCE-BASED/RELATIVE-VALUE SCALES

The principle of usual, reasonable, and customary fees for physician services was adopted with Medicare; subsequently, various forms of discounting and fee schedules have been tried. After prospective case-based pricing with DRGs was instituted for hospitals, the federal government looked for a mechanism to control the cost escalation under Medicare Part B for physician's services. They discussed DRGs for physicians, in use in Austria. The mechanism devised was resource-based/relative-value scales in which fees for physicians under Medicare Part B were set to reflect investments in training, years in practice, and regional cost of living. The underlying intent was to shift resources from specialties that emphasize technical and procedural services to those based on more cognitive problem solving for diagnosis and treatment—that is, from specialist to primary-care physicians. The formula for calculating the scales would have been extraordinarily cumbersome in the days before personal computers; indeed, the statistical manipulations are so complex that they provide a perfect screen for the real purpose—rigid and controlled fee schedules.

THERAPEUTIC PROTOCOLS

Practice guidelines are being developed for specific diagnoses and disease states.[6] The goal is to characterize exemplary patient care and to explore options in terms of costs and benefits. The assumption is that practice guidelines for appropriate utilization of services can improve the quality of care and reduce unit costs. Looking into the future, I call practice guidelines therapeutic protocols.

I call these six instruments for cost containment the Lilliputian scenario (see fig. 5). Like Captain Lemuel Gulliver, the ship's surgeon on *The Swallow*, modern-day physicians are bound by an army of Lilliputians. What binds the Gullivers of today is the red tape of prior authorization, second opinion, utilization review, diagnostic-related groups, resource-based/relative-value scales, and therapeutic protocols. Physicians have learned that if you have enough red tape you have enough rope to hang yourself.

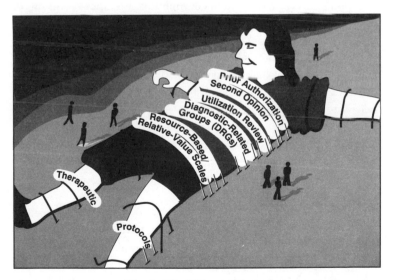

Fig. 5. The Lilliputian Scenario

From Myth to Reality

John Watkins, professor of pediatrics at the Children's Hospital of Philadelphia, has treated a young boy with a rare immunodeficiency. Lifesaving treatments with gamma globulin cost $97,000 per year, almost four times the average per capita income in the United States. This dramatic clinical circumstance illustrates the downside of medical miracles. Radical chemotherapy with bone-marrow transplantation is increasingly being tested in a variety of cancers, including lymphomas, leukemias, and carcinoma of the breast. The cost per treatment for this sophisticated technology totals approximately $150,000 to $200,000. Who will decide the therapeutic feasibility and the payment responsibility?

Thirty percent of expenditures by Medicare Part A are for patients in the last year of life.[7] The disproportionate allocation of health resources near the end of life—rather than more gradual allocation across the life span—is a dramatic example of the "no cost is too great" strategy. Community-based home-care hospice programs have demonstrated a cost-effective alternative for terminally ill cancer patients. Comprehensive-care retirement communities attempt to focus on the final years of living rather than on the months of dying.[8] Hundreds of billions of dollars are at stake.

When, early in the 1960s, the United States was devoting approximately 6 percent of the gross domestic product to health and medical care for a population of less than 200 million Americans, policy makers believed that universal access could be achieved as social policy with a few more percentage points of GDP. Sweden, where health planners advocated 10 percent of societal resources, was often cited as a prototype. Universal access meant the availability of the highest-quality health care for all. Resource allocation to achieve cost-effectiveness was discussed.

Rationing, unthinkable in the early 1960s, is now a compelling reality. Rationing health care means that not everyone can have complete access to the highest-quality health care available. One death, it is said, is a tragedy; a thousand deaths are a statistic. In health-care rationing, some of our statistics are destined to be recorded as tragic deaths.

The upper limits of resource allocation for health care ultimately derive from the competing needs within society. Health care cannot claim a predetermined portion of the gross domestic product. Other economically competitive societies now spend between 8 and 10 percent of GDP, while the United States is enroute to 18 or 19 percent by the year 2000.[9] The United States will then be spending three times as much on health care as on education.

The strategies for balancing needs and resources include increasing available resources, reducing need, selecting patients and treatment modalities, and realizing cost-effectiveness. Throughout the 1960s, 1970s, and 1980s, the United States sought to increase resources; now it is time to address the other strategies. The following eight mechanisms for resource allocation illustrate the boundaries and dimensions of the choices that must be made. They are not mutually exclusive; rather they can be adapted in various settings and among individual populations. But the institution specifying the benefits controls the analysis.

PREVENTION TO REDUCE NEED

Health promotion and disease prevention are obvious areas for anticipatory strategies. Pre- and postnatal care is only the beginning. Infant and childhood immunizations are classic priorities that cannot be left to passive, reactive strategies, neither can many of the health-promotion and disease-prevention priorities in the workforce, such as reducing occupational hazards; detecting and treating hypertension; eliminating cigarette smoking, excessive alcohol consumption, and drunk driving; and encouraging dietary prudence. Eternal vigilance is the price of disease prevention, and even reaching old age merely shifts one's priorities.

"Disease lies with the host" is an axiom of epidemiology; "and so does its treatment" should follow. Behavior modification and disciplined adherence to prescribed therapy have been very effective in reducing the incidence of stroke, for one. The broader lesson lies in the partnership of physician and patient in prevention, health promotion, and primary care. Resources invested in screening, detection, and early treatment of life-threatening diseases such as cancer of the breast, cervix, and colon can eliminate later expenditures for radical procedures, prolonged hospitalization, and palliative care.

The health behavior of a prospective mother has a greater impact on the delivery of a healthy infant than does the biomedical technology of amniocentesis, sonograms, and fetal monitoring. Prenatal care, supervision of labor, and the services of an obstetrician or nurse-midwife are important; this intervention, however, totals less than one day (a dozen fifteen- to thirty-minute office visits and a twelve- to eighteen-hour labor on average)—a mere fraction of a 270-day pregnancy. The patient needs education and counseling. Prospective rather than reactive strategies are required.

Not all prevention is low-cost and high-payoff.[10] One must always consider the costs of false positives—for example, a misleading cardiac stress test that leads to angiography and conceivably open-heart surgery. Colonoscopy, although superior to detection of occult blood, flexible sigmoidoscopy, or barium enema in identifying precancerous polyps, can cost up to $1,700 per procedure; a positive yield of 3 percent would result in a cost of $60,000 per polyp detected. Prevention may also pit infinite needs against finite resources.

CLINICAL SUITABILITY

The mechanism of clinical suitability assumes that the physician is the best judge of which resources to use to achieve desirable outcomes. Two factors—technology and the patient's condition—influence the physician. Physicians confront questions of clinical suitability for a variety of conditions. To determine clinical eligibility, the Medicare hospice benefit requires the physician to certify that the patient has less than six months to live. The neonatal intensive-care unit provides a forum in which issues of biomedical science, economics, and ethics are played out daily. Survival probabilities, long-term prognoses, and costs are all part of the equation. There is also the question of how much the individual will benefit—and how much relative to other potential patients. Medicine continues its search for scientific answers to these problems. One system, Acute Physiology and Chronic Health Evaluation (APACHE), uses quantitative methodology to predict outcomes in intensive-care units and thereby determine the probabilities of who will live and for how long. It could well become a basis for resource allocation by clinical suitability.

The work of J. E. Wennberg and his colleagues at the Center for the Evaluative Clinical Sciences at Dartmouth Medical School addresses the issue of professional conviction as to clinical suitability. It seems that communities vary widely in the prevalence of certain surgical procedures (see table 6).[11] One has about twice the likelihood of having a coronary artery bypass graft (open-heart surgery) in Rochester, N.Y., Orlando, or Iowa City as one does in Springfield, Mass. The probability of back and neck surgery in Orlando is about half that in Springfield and Tucson, and in Iowa City the probability is similarly small. Expectant mothers in Iowa City have a much higher probability of delivering a newborn vaginally than do their counterparts in Tallahasee and Orlando. These regional variations in utilization of health services give no clue as to which level is appropriate. The data reveal differences in physicians' judgments as to clinical suitability.

RATIONING BY THE BODY POLITIC

Decision making is sometimes broadened beyond physicians to incorporate the entire electorate. In Oregon, for example, citizens

Table 6
Regional Variations in Incidence of Surgery

	Coronary Artery Bypass Graft[a]	Caesarean	Back and Neck[a]
Seattle, Wash.	9.1	18.5%	12.8
Sacramento, Calif.	9.6	20.4%	14.2
Tucson, Ariz.	6.5	21.0%	16.2
Iowa City, Iowa	15.3	13.5%	9.4
Tallahassee, Fla.	8.2	28.8%	13.1
Orlando, Fla.	11.1	28.3%	8.3
Springfield, Mass.	6.0	25.7%	19.2
Rochester, N.Y.	11.0	20.6%	12.6

[a]Number per 10,000 residents

evaluated 1,600 clinical conditions to determine priorities for utilization of finite resources. Through public referendum, Oregon has sought to define an affordable level of basic health services for Medicaid recipients. Basic services include health promotion and disease prevention, primary care, and secondary services available in community hospitals. Trade-offs are being made between questionable tertiary care for a few and primary care for many. I discuss this issue in chapter 9.

WAITING TIME

Many industrially developed societies use waiting time as a mechanism for resource allocation. "Queuing," an essential characteristic of the British National Health Service, is a mechanism of resource allocation between the general practitioner and hospital-based specialists. Interestingly, patients in the United Kingdom do not think of health services as rationed; rather they think of themselves as waiting their turns.

While a wait of three years for an elective hernia repair in the United Kingdom might be acceptable, next week can be considered an unusually long time to wait for an MRI in the United States. For selected diagnostic studies or therapeutic procedures in nonemergency conditions, a wait of two days or a week would not seem to diminish quality significantly. Can, or rather will, Americans wait for referral from primary and secondary care to medical centers offering expensive tertiary care? Waiting may, after all, be the most effective technique for balancing infinite needs and finite resources.

CLINICAL TRIALS

The testing of newly developed drugs entails extensive clinical trials to determine their safety and efficacy. With many medications and therapeutic procedures the clinical trial remains equivocal. The more experience with a medication or procedure, the more frequently untoward side effects that require evaluation are detected. With some therapeutic strategies, more extensive and sophisticated clinical trials are carried out, and the results contradict earlier findings.

For much advanced biomedical technology, application never really moves beyond clinical trials. Thus their widespread use could yield a mechanism for resource allocation. Utilization of such technology could be approached as part of ongoing clinical trials contrasting the latest technology with that already existing.

Clinical-outcomes research speaks to this issue. Recognizing most tertiary care as an ongoing clinical trial could contribute to meaningful allocation of resources among different strategies. When we refer to the "practice" of medicine, we imply a constant search for better performance. The clinical trial is such a strategy.

The clinical trial is often a random-control trial in which allocation to the experimental or control group is determined by chance. If one has equity as the objective, random selection fills the bill. If tertiary care, for example, is viewed as a clinical trial, the element of randomness introduced offers greater equity than now exists.

ADMISSIONS COMMITTEES

We are accustomed to the role of the admissions committee in our society. Admission standards represent the allocation of a scarce resource. In the early days of chronic renal dialysis, anonymous committees established priorities for determining which patients would receive the treatment. Transplantation teams, too, are de facto admissions committees allocating scarce resources. The process combines scientific judgment with subjective decisions; its pros and cons need to be better understood.

HEALTH-SERVICES LOTTERY

The Pennsylvania lottery benefits senior citizens. Why not have a health-care lottery for tertiary care? In many ways it would be an extension of catastrophic health insurance except that, instead of adjusted premiums to cover anticipated risk, premiums would be constant through the ticket price and the coverage would be variable.

PROSPECTIVE BUDGET

On less than a societal scale, health-care systems have budgetary control of expenditures. Group Health Cooperative of Puget Sound in Seattle, Washington, a staff-model health maintenance organization, for example, must address the health-care needs of 480,000 subscribers with an annual budget of approximately $850 million.[12] Like Oregon, Group Health confronts the issue of finite resources by addressing the needs of the population at risk. Using its subscribers as well as its providers to develop health-care strategies, Group Health seeks cost-effective approximations.

The board of Group Health can decide to increase premiums and therefore income, but it risks losing subscribers to alternative delivery systems in the Washington-Oregon area. It could decide instead to cut back on basic services or to alter the mix of services within projected income. These are all available strategies for maintaining a cost-effective program.

What does such an organization, working with a fixed income, do about a problem like breast cancer? The disease can be approached through screening based on self-examination (which can be taught), examination by nurse practitioners or physicians (either generalists or specialists), and/or mammography. If a lesion is detected, options include lumpectomy, segmental resection, and mastectomy, which may or may not be followed by chemotherapy and radiation. Can early detection and intervention substitute for more radical and costly treatment later? Certainly this strategy has clinical benefits for the patient, as well as financial advantages for the health maintenance organization.

In deciding what combination of resource consumption offers the best probability for desired outcomes, systems will be able to draw increasingly on the work of national consensus panels in various areas of technology assessment. Ultimately, however, the decisions are judgment calls. Heretofore they have been made by the physician and other health professionals; now the arena is being enlarged to incorporate patients and institutions. Given the pluralism of American society, the decisions will be complex and multifaceted.

I advocate health-care delivery systems that follow the example of

Group Health Cooperative of Puget Sound and other HMOs. The budget that is prospectively allocated on an annual basis is derived from the capitation payments of enrolled subscribers rather than from a central appropriation from government. The more widespread the participation in decision making for resource allocation, the greater the acceptance by and effectiveness for the patient and the health-care professional. The next chapter examines the characteristics of health-care systems.

Chapter 6
Medicine and Management

Health-care systems are a
paradigm for our time.

Cost-effective health care requires the informed and intensive collaboration of medicine and management.[1] Unfortunately, they
tend to view the health-care enterprise very differently. To physicians,
the essence is individual physician-patient encounters, patient hospital days, nurse-patient contact hours, diagnoses, and procedures. To
managers, the $1 trillion-plus colossus called health care is a challenge
to corporate practices of finance, accounting, organization, planning,
and personnel. The efforts of these two cultures to face medicine's
dilemmas can result in conflict and confrontation—or in collaboration
and synthesis.

Traditionally, medicine—or, more precisely, physicians—had the
upper hand. Hospital administrations looked to their boards of
trustees for operational and budget decisions and then hired nurses
and other staff. The physician, as a member of a voluntary hospital
staff, enjoyed the privileges of admitting patients and allocating the
hospital's resources. The system, not the most efficient or effective
according to the principles of management, worked because third par-

ties picked up the tab through a system of open-ended financing based on retrospective cost-based reimbursement.

The ascendancy of the administrator, now the president and CEO, has been shaped by financing. The large influx of funds when Medicare joined the third parties offered the opportunity to expand administrative staffs, and prospective case-based pricing using diagnostic-related groups meant the physician on the voluntary staff became less of a free agent and more of a team player. His or her behavior and a hospital's financial survival were now locked together. The hospital president and CEO became responsible for operations, budgets, and—most of all—personnel, as hospitals are labor-intensive industries.

Table 7 summarizes the contrasting concerns and mechanisms of medicine and management. Medicine emphasizes personal responsibility for the care of the patient; management emphasizes delegation of authority and responsibility. Medical care in the United States emphasizes the specialist; management requires the abilities of the generalist. The medical practitioner is compelled to master a body of knowledge to ensure expertise; the manager, by contrast, is trained to orchestrate the expertise of others. The physician treats disease at any cost; management must address resource allocation and limitations. While physicians deal with individuals or families, management deals with consumers aggregated into markets. One of the most distinctive

Table 7
The Contrasts between Medicine and Management

Medicine	Management
Personal responsibility	Delegation
Specialists	Generalists
Possession of expertise	Orchestration of expertise
No cost too great	Resource limitations
Individuals (patients)	Markets (consumers)
Reactive	Anticipatory
Authoritative	Entrepreneurial
Professional standards	Consumer perceptions
Accreditation, licensure, certification	Job description
Income targeters	Income maximizers
Independent practice	Group process

contrasts between medicine and management is the character of initiatives. Medicine is reactive, while management is anticipatory. The physician stands ready to provide the highest-quality health care when consulted by the patient. The manager is concerned with the proactive determination of priorities.

Management seeks gains at the margin through productivity; medicine pursues precision in diagnosis and treatment. For the physician, quality is predominantly determined by professional judgment, while the manager perceives it as determined by the evaluations of diverse stakeholders. The manager faces competition from newly emerging entities entering markets. The physician is protected by accreditation, licensure, and specialty certification. In the corporate sector, positions are defined by job descriptions and then filled; the physician with a specialty designation carries the job description from setting to setting. Managers are presumed to be income maximizers, always reaching for new levels of revenues or income. Physicians are income targeters seeking a comfortable (that is, very comfortable) income and then trading off additional income for leisure time or preferred pursuits. Medicine is an endeavor driven by solo practitioners' interests and aspirations. Management is a group process.

Reconciling these differences can mean quality medical care delivered in a cost-effective fashion. Pragmatic and pluralistic health-care systems are the American way to realize cost-effective services. Although Americans have tended to prefer informal, loose systems, they will soon be compelled to accept intensely interdependent organizations. Increasingly, organized medicine, traditionally a descriptive term for the American Medical Association, will connote systems designed to provide comprehensive health services for defined populations.

The corporation is the dominant vehicle in American society for organizing resources to produce goods and services. Health-care systems represent the corporate structure and strategy for the organization, financing, and delivery of health services. Corporations seek to provide goods or services for consumers in preferred markets. Health-care systems address the consumer, or patient, as an individual within an enrolled population.

The corporate practice of medicine is a concept that has long been anathema to the American Medical Association, whose crusade against it began in state legislatures after World War II. The experiences of thousands of physicians who had been drafted into the military and subjected to the workings of a large bureaucracy no doubt contributed to the widespread suspicion of corporate practice. Nevertheless, it is a concept that evolved over the ensuing years until the introduction of health maintenance organizations in the 1970s.

In *The Social Transformation of American Medicine*, Paul Starr announces "the coming of the corporation," and Arnold S. Relman, former editor of the *New England Journal of Medicine*, speaks of "the new medical-industrial complex."[2] The health-care version of corporate production functions and entrepreneurial factors is represented by delivery systems distinguished by various financial mechanisms and patterns of organization. The governance and management of health-care systems provide the direction to make them purposeful and effective in meeting population needs, and the variation in values, priorities, size, and scope is extensive. The components and interrelations in health-care systems are diagrammed in figure 6.

The resources in health-care systems are largely unique—biotechnology, hospitals, physicians, nurses, and other health person-

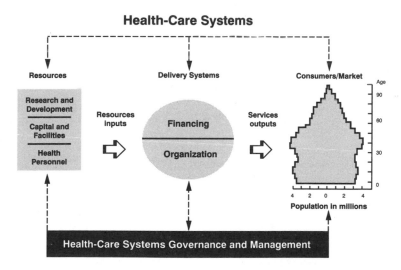

Health-Care Systems

Fig. 6. The Components and Interrelations in Health-Care Systems

nel. Changes associated with one resource invariably precipitate developments in another. Biomedical advances, for example, have changed the character of medical practice, and the availability of certain medical specialties influences the utilization of services they provide. Reciprocally, shortages of primary-care physicians have meant that medical specialists have provided primary care, often in an inappropriate manner. The utilization of basic resource inputs is shaped by mechanisms of financing and patterns of organization: while fee for service and retrospective cost-based reimbursement represent forceful incentives for increased services, capitation and prospective budgets tend to limit the utilization of resource inputs. The financing mechanisms and patterns of organization in delivery systems can provide a significant force for the realization of cost-effective health services.

The major distinction between corporations and health-care systems is in their governance and management. Corporations are hierarchical in the accountability of the executive leadership to the board of directors and shareholders. In health-care systems, governance and management tend to be more collegial and collaborative. Although the systems encompass sophisticated scientific knowledge, highly trained professionals, elaborate facilities, and costly state-of-the-art technology, the essential ingredient in health care remains a personal interaction—between a physician and a patient or a patient and a nurse. Dentists, pharmacists, optometrists, physical therapists, social workers, and other health professionals expand the boundaries and dimensions of health care. It is a social endeavor comprising billions of interactions annually.

But the American corporation is evolving. Increasingly, accountability is being viewed as an obligation owed not just to shareholders but to "stakeholders," a group that includes more than merely those who own stock in the corporation. The needs and expectations of these diverse stakeholders—suppliers, communities, governments, and consumers—have meant that CEOs focus more and more on the outside environment and rely on chief operating officers for internal management.

Can health-care systems be far behind? The stakeholders of health-care systems are diverse and powerful. Moreover, the health-care CEO presides over a similarly varied constituency. The classic levers of corporate management, such as accounting, are less useful than communication, negotiation, and persuasion skills. The health-care systems model suggests a negotiated relationship between the provider and the patient, or subscriber. The dual accountability to stakeholders will be increasingly political in the coming era of resource allocation and rationing. Indeed, the twenty-first century will likely see a transition from the management model to the political model of institutional leadership. The CEO will be less a president and more a prime minister, leading multiple constituents and fully recognizing that in addition to electoral renewal by a board one must be ever ready to win a vote of confidence from one's peers.

Like planning and management in health care, governance has evolved in recent decades from an informal process, chiefly in hospitals, to one concerned with disciplined corporate budgeting and financial accountability. Once managers were called superintendents or administrators and were responsible for attending to details, not creating strategies; boards of trustees characteristically took their lead from medical staffs composed of physicians on voluntary appointment. At trustee meetings it was not unusual to hear the question, "What do the doctors want?" The emergence of health care from a sovereign profession, however, has had far-reaching implications for governance. The yielding of the Marcus Welby scenario to health-care systems is altering the authority, autonomy, and prerogative of the physician, who is being transformed from a solo player to a team player. Trustees, in turn, are increasingly shouldering their fiduciary accountability for the institutions—composed of nurses, managers, technicians, as well as physicians—that serve patients.

Although predominantly voluntary and not-for-profit, health-care systems can be grouped in the following categories: entrepreneurial, eleemosynary, ecclesiastical, elected. Entrepreneurial systems compete for capital in equity markets. Eleemosynary, or charitable, not-for-profit institutions include most voluntary community hospitals. Ecclesiastical institutions are a variation accountable to religious authority as well as to the community. Institutions in the public sector—those managed by the federal government or operated as state or municipal hospitals—are accountable to the electorate and are therefore called elected. While values, goals, and missions vary, the delivery of medical care to the patient can be almost identical across institutions.

No two health-care systems are alike. A small health center such as the Lincoln County Primary Care Center in Hamlin, West Virginia, contrasts with the Henry Ford Health System in Detroit. On an even larger scale, health-care systems are represented by the Kaiser Foundation Health Plan, with 9,000 physicians responsible for 6.6 million enrollees and a budget of $11 billion in 1992, or the Department of Medicine and Surgery of the Veterans Administration.

The allocation of hundreds of billions of dollars for health care uses markets, regulation, government, and often a complex combination of all three. And not surprisingly, every special interest in American society has a position of advocacy on health policy. The adaptation, modification, and implementation of policy, therefore, is pursued by multiple institutions and individuals operating separately but usually interacting in the private, independent, and public sectors. Such participation in the shaping and implementation of societal priorities constitutes what Gunnar Myrdal calls the "institutional infrastructure of modern organized society"; public policy, he observes, "is now decided upon and executed in many different sectors and on different levels."[3]

The infrastructure in health care is the organization and arrangement of constituents that are supportive of the endeavor. Most of the health-care enterprise attempts to synthesize private- and public-sector initiatives and accountability; it is the interaction of these sectors with each other and with national policy considerations that contributes to the institutional infrastructure shown in figure 7. In the center are the prototypical health-care systems, representing thousands of organizations and institutions. They can be said to be embedded in the institutional infrastructure. The pluralism of health policy from the national perspective is shown in the diagram both by government policy and programs and by voluntary and private-sector initiatives. Prospective payment by diagnostic-related groups and resource-based/relative-value scales are illustrations of government policy and programs. The Joint Commission on Accreditation of Healthcare Organizations; managed-care initiatives of Aetna, CIGNA, and Prudential; and the Liaison Committee on Medical Education for the accreditation of schools of medicine are examples of voluntary and private-sector initiatives.[4]

These national initiatives interact with health-care institutions in

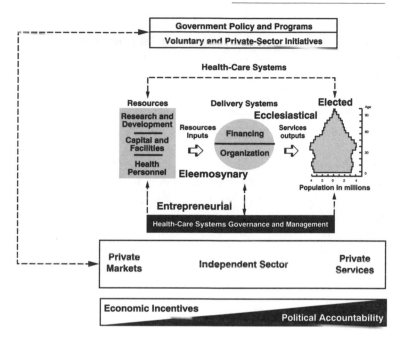

Fig. 7. The Health-Care Enterprise

private markets, the independent sector, and public services. The majority of health-care initiatives are in the independent sector; public services represent a third and private markets a tenth. These latter two health-care institutions are influenced mainly by political accountability and economic incentives respectively in the infrastructure.

Health policy reflects constant evolution as the society seeks to develop optimal incentives for, and constraints on, physicians, nurses, hospitals, insurers, patients, and other stakeholders in health affairs. Some initiatives, such as licensure, accreditation, and certification, span a century; other modifications, such as prospective case-based payment with diagnostic-related groups and resource-based/relative-value scales emerged during the 1980s. Health-care systems now seek to define a middle ground of nongovernmental community responsibility in the public interest: a social utility, a quasi-governmental organization, or a franchised service with governmental standards and regulation.

The health-care enterprise can readily be seen as a sovereign profession when measured by its advocacy of the patient, professional accountability, and compassionate care. But it is also a vast industry if measured by its numbers of physicians, nurses, hospitals, nursing homes, pharmaceuticals, and insurance companies and by the staggering magnitude of its technology. As we deal with the health-care enterprise of the future, it is incumbent on us to recognize when we measure it as a profession and when as an industry. Any attempted change in the industry will affect the profession, and vice versa.

Can the finest principles and practices of medicine and management prevail in health care? Yes, if physicians, nurses, managers, and other health professionals appreciate the context within which they work—the dimensions, character, and requirements of health care and the challenges of infinite needs confronting finite resources.

Chapter 7
The Past as Prologue

Health policy is not created
on a clean canvas.

Until now, the United States has never undertaken a comprehensive legislative reform of health care comparable to the British
National Health Act of 1946. Even the two dozen health initiatives of
the Eighty-ninth Congress (1965–66) were less than all-encompassing.
The path, as described by Charles Lindblom, professor of political
science at Yale, has been one of incremental adjustments.[1] The health-
care enterprise, with its origins in colonial times and its precedents
imported from England, Scotland, and the Continent, has grown to
maturity largely since the 1930s.[2]

Contemporary health policy can best be understood in terms of six
sequential eras since then. The initial efforts toward a health policy
focused on population categories (1935–44), followed by resource development (1945–59), delivery systems (1960–69), institutional infrastructure (1970–79), and systems dynamics (1980–89). A sixth era,
concerned with values and priorities, began in the 1990s (see fig. 8).

The concept of comprehensive health services was addressed in
twenty-nine volumes published over five years by the Committee on

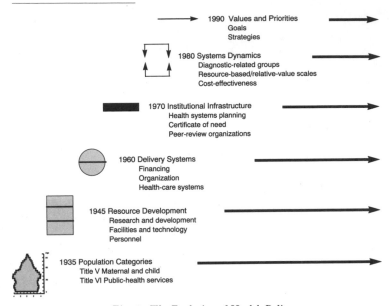

Fig. 8. The Evolution of Health Policy

the Costs of Medical Care, established in 1927 by a consortium of eight philanthropic foundations. Its final report, *Medical Care for the American People*, published in 1932, advanced the following recommendations:

1. Medical services, both preventive and therapeutic, should be furnished largely by organized groups of physicians, dentists, nurses, pharmacists, and other associated personnel.
2. All basic public-health services—whether provided by governmental or nongovernmental agencies—should be available to the entire population according to its needs.
3. The cost of medical care should be addressed on a group-payment basis, through the use of insurance and taxation.
4. Studies, evaluation, and coordination of medical services should be considered important functions for every state and local government.

5. The breadth, depth, and focus of education and
    training for the health professions should be expanded.

These recommendations, in whole or in part, have shaped the evolution of health policy for over half a century.

Population Categories (1935–44)

During the early 1930s, the Committee on Economic Security established by President Franklin D. Roosevelt was determined to address health care in proposed legislation.[4] Faced with vigorous opposition from the American Medical Association and with a political threat to Social Security, his prime domestic proposal, Roosevelt omitted the health-care provision from the final document.

The Social Security Act did, however, launch national health policy. The human misery experienced in the Great Depression dramatically demonstrated that voluntary efforts and the resources of state and local governments were insufficient to meet the health needs of the population. Health problems among the poor became so serious during the 1930s that the federal government was forced to become involved. The Federal Emergency Relief Administration was created in 1933 to provide states with grants-in-aid to maintain unemployment and relief programs.[5] Legislation was later expanded to provide some medical services to recipients of such programs.

Title V of the Social Security Act of 1935 authorized grants to individual states for maternal and child health programs. Title VI authorized annual appropriations "for the purpose of assisting states, counties, health districts and other political subdivisions of the states in establishing and maintaining adequate public health services."[6] Working through the states, in collaboration with local governments, Title V and Title VI focused on specialized problems (such as communicable-disease control) and special risk groups (such as women and children). They built on public-health and community initiatives going back to those of the Commonwealth of Massachusetts in 1869 and of the city of Baltimore in 1793.[7]

Consideration of health-insurance benefits for Social Security recipients, although dropped from Roosevelt's legislative proposal, was not abandoned. Deliberations continued. The National Health Bill introduced by Senator Robert F. Wagner, Democrat of New York, in 1939 led to the Wagner-Murray-Dingell proposals for national health insurance in the 1940s.[8] The outbreak of World War II had placed a moratorium on most domestic programs, so health care remained an individual concern to be addressed in the voluntary, or private, sector of society. The Wagner-Murray-Dingell bill was reintroduced three months after V-J Day. This version was drafted by Wilbur Cohen, later the principal architect of Medicare.

Resource Development (1945–59)

When President Harry S. Truman signed the Hospital Survey and Construction Act of 1946, widely known as the Hill-Burton program, he forecast the theme for national health policy that would prevail until the 1960s.[9] Although Truman proposed universal health insurance, the health-policy theme of the Fair Deal and of the ensuing Eisenhower administration was federal investment in resource development.[10]

Health and the services necessary to achieve it remained the private concern of individuals, except for those warranting public assistance. The federal government, however, undertook to ensure the availability of basic health resources. Priorities focused on the ingredients that gave health-service systems their character: research and development, facilities and technology, and personnel.

RESEARCH AND DEVELOPMENT

Congress showed its interest in medical research when it established the first of the National Institutes of Health, the National Cancer Institute, in 1937. Authorization of the National Heart Institute (now the National Heart, Blood, and Lung Institute) followed in 1948 and the National Institute of Mental Health in 1949. Other institutes were authorized in the 1950s, and today there are a dozen disease-specific national research institutes.

The strategy of the National Institutes of Health for support of undifferentiated and targeted research has been carried out on an unprecedented scale, so that investments have risen to almost $11 billion a year.[11] These investments have profoundly furthered knowledge of the biomedical aspects of disease, and they represent a clear commitment of tax resources in the interest of the public good.

FACILITIES AND TECHNOLOGY

Investments by the Hill-Burton program dramatically changed the character of health facilities in the United States. The program assisted more than 4,000 communities in building hospitals, public health centers, extended-care facilities, diagnostic and treatment centers, and rehabilitation facilities. In addition to supplying bricks and mortar, grants guided incorporation of technology, standards for care, and modifications in delivery systems.

The Hill-Burton program also fostered the development of area-wide hospital planning, although suggestions for extensive hospital planning were never executed.[12] Notwithstanding a bias toward rural areas in the distribution of grants, the initiatives sought to ensure that every community in the nation of any significant size had 4.5 general-hospital beds per 1,000 people.

PERSONNEL

Involvement of the federal government in the development of the health labor force began when the National Institute of Mental Health included support for the training of service, as well as research, personnel among its inaugural programs.[13] The next step was taken in 1956, when Congress authorized support for the training of public-health personnel to staff programs aided by Title VI of the Social Security Act. Initiatives in 1957 addressed training of nurses for administrative, supervisory, and teaching responsibilities. Although all these initiatives added a new dimension to national health policy, they represented only limited interests in the health labor force. Nonetheless, they created a momentum that carried forward for decades. Health-care reform in the twenty-first century must address many of the precedents and consequences.

Physicians for a Growing America, the 1959 report of the surgeon general's Consultant Group on Medical Education, argued for an expansion of medical schools to help maintain a ratio of 133 physicians per 100,000 population. The report launched federal support for the effort.[14] Four years later, a report by the surgeon general's Consultant Group on Nursing, identifying the need for 850,000 nurses and a feasible goal of 680,000, would similarly prompt legislation, the Nurse Training Act of 1964.[15] Investments in the development of health personnel would continue in the 1960s and 1970s with construction grants and student loans to schools of medicine and dentistry, the Health Professions Assistance Act amendments, the Allied Health Professions Personnel Training Act, and the omnibus Health Manpower Act.

Delivery Systems (1960–69)

It had long been assumed by Congress and the electorate that medical care was exclusively the business of physicians—that is, physicians made the purchasing decisions and someone else paid the bill. Throughout almost two decades of resource development, government assumed that if it invested sufficient funds in basic health resources the necessary services would be available to the general population. It became increasingly evident, however, that massive federal investments in resource development would not solve existing health problems. Despite the highest per capita expenditure in the world, health care in the United States offered neither adequate access nor the highest health status compared with that of other developed nations. The 1960s brought an end to complacency. In answer to mounting demands for solutions, the Kennedy and Johnson administrations and Congress led the society into a new era in health affairs.

The new theme in the 1960s was health-care delivery systems to make health services available and accessible to patients and populations. Although the strategy remained targeted rather than comprehensive, health-service delivery in the private, or voluntary, sector would no longer be free of government involvement. The congressional initiatives called for a "partnership" in the public interest.

Health policy continued to consider health care largely the private responsibility of the individual and the family. Public assistance for certain groups was expanded, however, and investments in financing, organization, and systems were added. The basic resources of knowledge, facilities, and personnel required an "entrepreneurial factor" or "production function" in order to translate into products or services.

The Social Security Amendments of 1965 were a landmark effort to eliminate economic barriers to medical care by extending coverage for the elderly and the medically indigent. Medicare and Medicaid, Titles XVIII and XIX of the amendments, expended billions of dollars on the status quo, paying usual, customary, and reasonable fees to physicians and reimbursing costs for hospital care. These two programs pumped money into an essentially nonmarket economy lacking checks, balances, and regulatory feedback. The laissez-faire strategy for financing persisted through the 1960s into the 1970s. The Nixon administration would try wage and price controls in 1971, reducing the rate of cost escalation for the short term but producing a rebound phenomenon that wiped out the savings and set costs back on a more rapidly rising trajectory. Efforts would follow to reshape the health-care enterprise through planning, competition, and regulatory infrastructures.

The Medicare and Medicaid legislation did not interfere with the existing practice of medicine. Congress effectively endorsed fee for service and solo practice as bulwarks against organizational change, but it did recognize financial and organizational strategies. Although Medicare and Medicaid chose to adopt the existing pattern of health services, other initiatives during the 1960s authorized grant support for programs that organized health services to serve population groups. These efforts evolved in the 1970s into health maintenance organizations, hospital-physician joint ventures, multi-institutional systems—now categorized as "alternative delivery systems"—and other health partnerships.[16]

The advances in organization were the result of seemingly unrelated legislative efforts targeting various segments of the population. The Migrant Health Act of 1962, a little-known initiative, was joined by the maternal and child health amendments of 1963, 1965, and 1967, which provided federal funds for the development of comprehensive health services. Creation of the Office of Economic Opportunity in 1964 led to more visible demonstration projects. Health centers and group practices were developed across the country for underserved and poverty-stricken communities. Although the dangers of two-class medical care—organized delivery systems for the poor and free-choice, solo-practice, and fee-for-service care for the middle class— were recognized, these OEO initiatives were soon followed by other programs.

The 1960s addressed organization as a subject more of experimentation than of implementation. Initiatives were on a small scale. The Partnership for Health authorized several project grants for development of programs providing comprehensive health services, including prepaid group practices such as the Harvard Community Health Plan and the Community Health Care Plan in New Haven, Connecticut, early prototypes of health maintenance organizations.[17] Although the lesser partner to financing, organization would eventually contribute to significant advances in the development of delivery systems.

Health policy, while moving across a broad front in the 1960s, did not attempt a comprehensive solution for meeting the health needs of the American people. The experiments in organization notwithstanding, the dominant conviction at the end of the 1960s continued to be that the health-care enterprise would work with tinkering rather than with an overhaul. Nevertheless, the agenda of the 1960s laid the groundwork for the Health Maintenance Organization Act of 1974. Since the end of World War II, medical societies had been successful in restricting group practice in more than forty states. When prepaid group practice was cloaked as "health maintenance organization" by consultants to the Department of Health, Education, and Welfare, however, Congress determined to interfere with the "established practice of physicians and hospitals" and enact legislation providing competitive alternatives to fee for service and to solo practice.[18] Contrasted with the aspirations of early HMO enthusiasts, subsequent developments have been rather slow.

Institutional Infrastructure (1970–79)

The dominant policy decisions of the 1970s affected the institutional infrastructure of the health-care enterprise. Diverse forces shape the institutional infrastructure of health affairs: national policies are decreed through the Health Care Financing Administration; voluntary initiatives may be advanced by the Blue Cross/Blue Shield Association or the American College of Physicians. Local communities and agencies in the public and private sectors shape the institutional infrastructure as well.

The regional medical programs and comprehensive health planning of the mid-1960s were way stations enroute to the National Health Planning and Resources Development Act of 1974. The imminent expiration of authorization for the Partnership for Health had provided Congress with an opportunity to reassess planning and regulatory mechanisms, and after extensive hearings the legislation was signed by President Gerald R. Ford in January 1975. A network of state health planning and development agencies and some 200 health systems agencies in communities throughout the nation, incorporating the state regulatory mechanism of certificate of need, sought "coordination of health services." This bold experiment failed and health planning declined, but many initiatives persist in business and health coalitions.

The Social Security Amendments of 1972 addressed the problems of cost and quality of medical care. The priority was clearly costs. The billions of dollars pumped into the health-care system since 1965 had fostered extraordinary inflation. Senator Wallace Bennett, Republican of Utah, proposed the creation of professional standards review organizations (PSROs) to assess the quality and costs of hospital services. The PSRO movement followed the rocky course that characterizes most new national programs. Although the PSROs were severely criticized for lack of cost-effectiveness, recent evidence indicates that they saved money by reducing unnecessary utilization. In 1982, PSROs were replaced as a regulatory measure by peer-review organizations (PROs).

The end of the 1970s saw the defeat of the hospital cost-containment legislation proposed by the Carter administration. The issues of planning and regulation had dominated a decade of health policy. Limits of intervention were still under debate. The Federal Trade Commission began to press the health-care enterprise to become more competitive and more responsive to market forces. It attacked a number of practices, from restrictions on physician advertising to physician domination of Blue Shield insurance boards. Such challenges reflected the conviction that the delivery of health care had to modify its reliance on physicians for decision making and avoid restraint of trade.

Systems Dynamics (1980–89)

All the components of systems were in place for the 1980s. The competitive and regulatory eclecticism of the health-care enterprise had contributed to a focus on systems dynamics. Perhaps nothing better illustrates these dynamics of interaction than diagnostic-related groups and resource-based/relative-value scales.

To some observers, DRGs are the central focus of competitive or market forces in health-care systems: hospitals ranging from small community institutions to major academic health centers compete, DRG by DRG, to produce competitive case mixes within prospective payment schedules. Other observers correctly point out that DRGs are in fact regulated prices for specific services and therefore eliminate price competition. As with much else in health care, the matter is one of perspective.

Resource-based/relative-value scales are another initiative of the federal government to regulate the economics of health-care delivery, this time by adopting a fee schedule that attempts to balance the cognitive and technical services provided by physicians. Technical procedures have been well compensated since the earlier days of Blue Shield, primarily because they are easy to count, measure, and price. Physicians' analyses, diagnoses, and consultations are another matter. Under the RB/RVS developed by William Hsiao of the Harvard School of Public Health, the compensation of pediatricians and family physicians will rise at the expense of surgeons and radiologists. The result is a centralized effort to correct market imperfections.

The dynamics of health-care systems, as they emerged in the 1980s, represented a means to an end. The DRGs and RB/RVS call attention to the systems dynamics of an enterprise in which all the components are linked.

Values and Priorities (1990–)

Physician-patient interactions occur within the complex social system that is the health-care enterprise. Organization, financing, and delivery are all relevant concerns, as they are for other industries as well. The decades ahead will see a new focus on interrelations among the components and dimensions developed over five decades. The remainder of the twentieth century must be devoted to comprehending this enormous enterprise so as to discipline and direct it.

The past concerns of the American health-care system have been largely structural. Its future lies with goals and strategies. Decision making will be shaped not only by health professionals but increasingly by patients in their roles as consumers, clients, and constituents. What are some of the alternatives for effecting this change? The next chapter provides an overview of the major national health insurance proposals that will be influenced by these precedents.

Chapter 8
National Health Insurance

Health policy is tax policy.

Health-policy decisions are influenced by social, political, and economic circumstances external to health affairs per se. If one wishes to forecast health policy, one needs to keep an eye on the economy, the trade balance, unemployment, the savings and loan crisis, and the war against drugs, as well as on the AIDS epidemic, abortion conflicts, hospital mergers, health-care costs, and other subjects of today's headlines.

Like Medicare and Medicaid, health-care reform represents tax legislation. Medicare used two taxing mechanisms: Part A drew on employer and employee payroll deductions patterned after Social Security; Part B used general revenues to subsidize insurance premiums for physicians' fees. Medicaid drew on state appropriations derived from income tax, sales tax, and so forth and matched by general revenues from the federal government.

At present, close to $400 billion of health-care expenditures are provided by the public sector. Health-care reform could increase this amount significantly. Universal access and the core benefit package developed by the task force on health are projected to add $50 billion to $150 billion in annual expenditures. That is a challenge to any program of taxation. A value-added tax and taxes on payroll, health-insurance premiums, hospital charges, physicians' fees, prescriptions, cigarettes, and alcohol have all been discussed. While cost containment may reduce expenditures—or at least the rate at which expenditures rise—an increase in access and in benefits will require an increase in taxation, even if that taxation is called an employer-mandated contribution.

Proposed Legislation

Many thought national health insurance would come in the wake of Medicare. It did not. Yet a quarter-century later, when Harris Wofford defeated a favored opponent to retain his seat in the Senate, he launched the issue of access to health care. Health insurance and health-care reform became pivotal issues in the 1992 presidential election. George Bush supported market reform, while advisers to Bill Clinton began with a "play or pay" system and finished with managed competition, a synthesis of play or pay and managed care.

Since then, special-interest groups—the American Medical Association, American College of Physicians, American Nurses Association, National Council of Community Hospitals, and American Public Health Association, among others—have developed national health insurance policies. National health insurance or major health-care reform proposals introduced in the 103rd Congress have been predicated on single-payer, play-or-pay, or market-reform strategies or on a combination of them. Debates on national health insurance through the 1990s and into the twenty-first century will inevitably center on these themes.

SINGLE PAYER

A committee of more than 6,000 physicians headquartered in Cambridge, Massachusetts, advocates the single-payer approach as implemented in Canada.[1] The strategy would replace the current employer–private insurance health-care system with a publicly administered program not unlike Medicare or Medicaid. It could be funded through various forms of taxation.

Equity of access for all citizens is a priority of the Canadian system, which preserves solo practice and fee for service; cost containment is achieved through mandatory fee schedules for physicians and global budgeting (an annual limit on expenditures) imposed on hospitals. The elimination of commercial health insurance places the responsibility for billing and other paperwork with the government and thereby purportedly saves on administrative costs.

The single-payer strategy is particularly attractive for the implementation of cost containment. Once a health-care budget is set, however, the mechanisms for raising the funds must be addressed. In Canada the federal government has shifted budget responsibilities to the provinces, much as the American federal government mandates state services and leaves the states to generate tax revenues to pay for the programs. Allocating a budget among not just states but regions, communities, institutions, and individuals is another matter.

It seems unlikely that Congress will enact the single-payer approach as the sole mechanism of health-care financing. It would dramatically expand the administrative functions of government as well as the government's role in taxation. In addition, a number of stakeholders would adamantly oppose a single-payer system. The American health-insurance industry would fight the encroachment of government on a major market. Physicians and hospitals would fear control by an agency of the federal government. The public sector's portion of total expenditures would expand from the 42 percent represented by Medicare, Medicaid, and other public programs to two-thirds or more. Moreover, the probable utilization of Blue Cross, Blue Shield, and large commercial health insurers as fiscal intermediaries would undoubtedly undermine many of the savings and administrative costs lauded in the Canadian system.

Health-care recipients would not have to pay insurance premiums for services. A single-payer system could collect the equivalent of premiums through social insurance or taxation and allocate funds to physicians and hospitals on a negotiated-fee or contract basis. While the concept of single payer might be attractive because of its seeming simplicity, it runs the risk of implementing the mechanisms of payment before developing the innovations in delivery systems needed to provide cost-effective services. Canada has not been particularly prominent in health-systems innovation.

Canadian national health insurance builds on fee-for-service schedules negotiated between provincial governments and medical societies. Control of volume of services is another matter. The requisite cost containment in the United States would require relentless regulation—the Lilliputian scenario. Admittedly this problem also applies to other proposals for national health insurance.

PLAY OR PAY

The Bipartisan Commission on Comprehensive Health Care of the 101st Congress (1989–90) was originally chaired by Representative Claude Pepper, Democrat of Florida; at his death, he was succeeded by Senator John D. Rockefeller IV, Democrat of West Virginia. The Pepper Commission, composed of thirteen senators and representatives and three presidential appointees, formulated a carrot-and-stick strategy for health policy: the carrot consisted of financial incentives for reform while regulations and penalties constituted the stick.

The concept advocated—play or pay—would require all employers to either provide a basic package of health-insurance coverage for all employees or incur a 7 percent payroll tax. Not only large companies but also small businesses would be included. If they chose to pay the tax, their employees would be eligible for enrollment in a public program that would replace Medicaid for low-income citizens. This program would be funded through the tax on employers and companies that did not provide health insurance and a payroll tax on workers. Covered persons would also pay premiums up to 20 percent of costs based on their incomes. Those below the poverty level would be fully subsidized.

Play or pay—employer mandate to provide health insurance—builds on a long-standing tradition of employment-based third-party health insurance. It also dramatizes the differences between large employers and small businesses. The former command visibility; the latter provide the majority of jobs. Approximately ten percent of the work force are in firms of 1,000 or more employees; almost all of them have health insurance provided by their employers. Moreover, neither the employers nor the employees pay taxes on this benefit. Among firms with fewer than ten employees, only a quarter have health insurance provided by the employer. Play or pay, or employer mandate, has different implications for firms providing and those not providing health insurance: for the first group, the program means a new form of taxation; for the second, it means a conversion of a voluntary tax.

The program would be administered by the states, and payments would be overseen by state review boards. The boards would aim to reduce growth in health-care spending and set payment rates to be used by all payers or providers. A mandate for employers to purchase insurance cannot work unless insurance is more affordable. Proposals, therefore, usually call for community rating. Without adequate cost-control measures, play or pay could have a negative impact on small businesses, hitting employers with billions of dollars in new taxes.

MARKET REFORM

Proposals for market reform acknowledge that health affairs are extraordinarily diverse and complex, comprising federal, state, and local government initiatives; private-sector health insurance; and issues of autonomy and flexibility—all to serve a population representing extraordinary cultural pluralism. Market reforms emphasize tax credits, tax deductions, small-market insurance reform, and medical malpractice reform.

The key elements of the responsible national health insurance[2] proposal, initially utilized by the Bush administration for the 1992 campaign, include (1) a requirement that each citizen obtain minimum basic medical insurance adjusted inversely to family income; (2) fixed dollar tax credits or vouchers for families in need, including a full subsidy to cover health insurance premiums for poor families; (3) use of the federal tax system to collect net premiums for persons who did not purchase insurance; and (4) elimination of the subsidization of health insurance by including employer and employee contributions as taxable income. The proposal seeks to increase the availability, portability, and affordability of health insurance, particularly to small-business employers, their employees, and the dependents of those employees. The proposal became a very attractive vehicle for a variety of agendas, from small business insurance pools to simplification of administrative procedures and malpractice reform.

Current market-reform proposals recall the generous IRS deductions in the 1960s and 1970s for medical expenditures and health-insurance premiums but this time for the needy rather than the middle class. Further, the proposal assumes that once purchasing power is achieved the flow of funds will be guided by the forces of supply and demand in the market.

Performance Criteria

Single payer would replace the market. Play or pay would extend and enhance regulation of it. Market reform seeks to exploit it. Many proposals for national health insurance over the years did not resolve the tensions among cost, quality, and access. Each new proposal must face critical scrutiny from all sides.

The following criteria for analyzing national health insurance are adapted from those published in the *New England Journal of Medicine* in 1971 by Robert D. Eilers and ones published in 1992 by Marcia Angell.[3] The consistency of the criteria over two decades suggests that there is a consensus on what needs to be done. The question becomes how best to do it.

1. Universal Access

> Health care ought to be an entitlement for all
> Americans, with payment distributed equitably across
> the population rather than linked to one's ability to pay
> at time of service.

2. Comprehensiveness

Improvement in the health status of individuals and families, as well as of the population, requires a spectrum of health services, from health promotion and disease prevention to care by specialists and long-term care. National health insurance ought to support the development of a comprehensive continuum in health care over the span of an individual's lifetime.

3. Containment of Costs

Continued escalation of costs will ultimately provoke drastic countermeasures that could be detrimental to consumers as well as to providers. Health-care systems must be encouraged to seek cost-effectiveness and to contain costs.

4. Quality

Quality health care, as judged by professional, consumer, and community standards, must be encouraged by national health insurance. Maintaining high levels of satisfaction and morale for all parties requires no less.

5. Self-Regulation, Accountability, and Responsible Use of Services

The alternatives to being centrally managed are self-regulation and decentralized institutional accountability. Responsible utilization of services through effective provider and consumer collaboration in the determination of priorities is imperative.

If comprehensive services are seen as a dimension of quality, and self-regulation, accountability, and responsible use of services are yoked under cost containment, it is clear once again that what must be confronted are the tensions of access, quality, and cost containment.

The Eilers-Angell criteria, therefore, provide a good frame of reference for comparing the proposals for national health insurance. None of the three categories of proposed national health insurance addresses all the criteria equally. Nor do they address them in the same way.

SINGLE PAYER

1. Universal access is sought by providing public financing for everyone and eliminating a role for private, voluntary health insurance.
2. Comprehensive health services continue existing patterns of practice: free choice of physicians and hospitals.
3. Cost containment is achieved primarily through a fee schedule for all physicians and prospective budgeting for hospitals. Government financing and administrative procedures substitute for those of independent and competitive insurance companies.
4. Quality of care relies on traditional mechanisms of licensure, certification, accreditation, and promulgated standards.
5. Self-regulation, accountability, and responsible use of services rely on government-operated regulatory strategies for direct public sector control of the flow of dollars throughout the system. The consumer has very little role in the cost of health care.

PLAY OR PAY

1. Universal access is sought through employer-mandated benefits and public programs.
2. Comprehensive health services are addressed more by financing than by alternatives in delivery systems.
3. Increased consumer awareness on the part of employees will be stimulated by sharing of costs for premiums.

Funding of the health plans through payroll deductions and taxes tend, of course, to obscure cost sharing.

4. Quality of care relies on state review, development of national practice guidelines, implementation of a national uniform data system, research and development on quality assurance and assessment, federal standards, audits, certification, and research on quality-enhancement strategies.

5. Self-regulation, accountability, and responsible use of services are addressed by governmental oversight and efforts to extend the federal strategy of Medicare and the state strategy of Medicaid for significant governmental regulation.

MARKET REFORM

1. Universal access is sought through tax credits and deductions that enable individuals to purchase health insurance.

2. Comprehensive health services involve no modifications in delivery systems beyond improving the information base used in consumer selection.

3. Cost containment relies primarily on the market. There is little to influence a restructuring of health-care services so as to reduce costs or increase cost-effectiveness.

4. Quality of care is assumed to be inherent in the market, and the principle of caveat emptor prevails. Educated consumers would be put to the test.

5. Self-regulation, accountability, and responsible use of services are represented by limited intervention in the organization, financing, and delivery of health services. The question is the degree to which there will be tinkering with markets through regulation in order to achieve cost containment. Of the different proposals,

the market model relies most extensively on consumer participation in cost control and the pursuit of cost-effectiveness.

Policy proponents work to convince their audiences that their proposals can meet everyone's needs. Realistically, no national health-insurance scheme will meet all the needs and priorities of every consumer, provider, or community all of the time. Use table 8 as a score-card for evaluating the proposals. Each strategy can be scored from 10 (highest) to 1 (lowest) for each of the various criteria. Your total scores will suggest your preferences among the proposals. The matrix can, of course, be expanded to include additional specific proposals (A, B, and C in the table) so you can compare evaluations in the months to come.

Managed Competition

During the deliberations of President Johnson's task force, the chairman, Dr. George James, commissioner of health for New

Table 8
National Health Insurance

Performance Criteria	Alternative Proposals					
	Single Payer	Play or Pay	Market Reform	A	B	C
Universal Access						
Comprehensive Services						
Cost Containment						
Quality						
Self-Regulation, Accountability, and Responsible Use of Services						
Total						

York City, expressed his conviction that financing health care without restructuring would lead to severe cost escalation. Three decades of experience with Medicare and Medicaid have proved him correct.

Organizing and delivering health services is even more complex and emotionally charged than financing them. The Great Society health programs included only modest initiatives; organization of health services did not begin to develop as a partner to financing until the HMO Act of 1974. Health-care reform is now addressing patterns of organization as well as financing mechanisms.

A consumer-choice health plan, the conceptual forerunner of managed competition, has been refined for almost two decades by Alain Enthoven, professor of management at the Stanford University School of Business.[4] He proposes a combination of market forces, incentives to employers, and public subsidies to foster competition among health-care delivery systems in the form of centralized and decentralized health maintenance organizations, preferred provider organizations, and provider networks. The individual or group of consumers is encouraged to express preferences for health-services priorities within community and regional systems. As an economist, Enthoven makes it clear that he does not presume to know what is best for each individual but seeks to interpret the costs and implications of the alternatives.

In managed competition, accountable health partnerships resembling a consortium of health maintenance organizations, preferred provider organizations, and hospital-physician joint ventures would serve enrolled populations of up to several hundred thousand subscribers. Approximately 40 million Americans—more than 15 percent of the population—are enrolled in some 550 HMOs at present.

Health alliances, or health-insurance purchasing cooperatives— the second component—are fiscal intermediaries that pool enrollees and purchasing power so as to broker and negotiate with health plans. The alliances have precedent in the health-benefits program for federal employees. Five years before Congress authorized Medicare, federal employees could choose indemnity (a commercial carrier like Aetna), comprehensive benefits (Blue Cross/Blue Shield), or prepaid group practice (Kaiser Permanente or Health Insurance Plan of Greater New York). Each of 325 plans is subsidized at the same level by the federal government, and the employee is responsible for the different premium. Costs are contained for the government; the employee has to determine tradeoffs of access and quality. The program covers almost 10 million federal employees; a 26-fold expansion to the full population would be a challenge to implement. Medicare fiscal intermediaries across the country could serve as prototypes.

A third element—a National Health Board patterned after the Federal Reserve Board—is proposed. Responsibilities would include determination of the core package of health benefits, budgets, resource allocation, premiums, quality standards, reporting requirements, consumer and provider satisfaction, outcomes, health-service priority, and cost of services. Many of the proposed functions of a National Health Board are already under way in the Health Care Financing Administration, the National Institutes of Health, and the Agency for Health Care Policy and Research. Incorporating new functions could well be more effective than creating yet another federal bureaucracy. Moreover, initiatives in total quality management, cost-effectiveness, and continuous quality improvement are rapidly becoming all-pervasive throughout the American health-care enterprise. A National Health Board could well inhibit and constrain rather than promote reform.

A global budget is a fourth element some proponents have added to managed competition. Most analysts of health-care financing conclude that expenditures of 14 percent of GDP (and a projected 18 or 19 percent) are out of line with the 8 to 10 percent expenditures of America's economic competitors. How can costs be contained? Will market forces, abetted by fiscal and tax policy, do the trick, or will more regulation through fee schedules, premium caps, utilization controls, or wage and price controls be required? Once begun, where should efforts to regulate the world's eighth-largest economy stop? Managed competition, suggesting negotiations between monopsony purchasers and quasi monopoly providers is an all-pervasive, yet untested, theory. The interrelationships among and between the four main elements of health-care reform await definition, measurement, and testing.

Successful implementation of managed competition will call for effective negotiation between the purchasers (health alliances and independent buyers acting as such) and health-care systems (accountable health plans). The iron triangle of health care will be at the center of these negotiations. How will all this be paid for? How, in other words, can financing mechanisms be adapted to a new organization and delivery of services across the spectrum of health promotion, disease prevention, primary care, and specialized services? We will all pay, of course—not usually at the time of service but through a variety of overt and covert mechanisms. Who pays how much to benefit whom? A national health policy is a tax policy. Taxation, cross-subsidization, cost shifting, and benefits in lieu of wages are all issues to be deliberated. The bottom line will always be the same: balancing the tensions among access, quality, and cost containment. A glance at the issues on Capitol Hill should help make that clear.

Health-Care Reform and the 103rd Congress

President Clinton and Hillary Rodham Clinton delivered the *Health Security Act*, to Capitol Hill on Wednesday, 27 October 1993. The bill was introduced as S.R. 1757 by George Mitchell, majority leader of the Senate, and (on 20 November) as H.R. 3600 by Representative Richard Gephardt, majority leader of the House, with thirty cosponsors in the Senate and some one hundred in the House. It joined several other initiatives.

The *American Health Security Act* (S.R. 491) was introduced by Senator Paul D. Wellstone, Democrat of Minnesota, and Representative Jim McDermott of Washington (H.R. 1200) on 3 March 1993. The proposal would provide universal access to a generous benefit package, utilizing government financing of a single payer program through payroll taxes and state administration. Annual budgets would require negotiation of physician fees or capitation and hospital payments. Medicare and Medicaid would be phased in. Insurance companies could provide supplemental coverage and serve as fiscal intermediaries. This proposal also has almost one hundred cosponsors in the House.

Representative Fortney "Pete" Stark of California, the chairman of the health subcommittee of House Ways and Means introduced the Mediplan Health Care Act (H.R. 2610) on 1 July 1993. The act would extend Medicare benefits to the entire population. Existing Medicare payment mechanisms (e.g., DRGS and RB/RVSS) or capitation for HMOS would be used to achieve a global budget. Financing of premiums would be 80 percent employer and 20 percent employee. Insurance companies would be limited to fiscal intermediary roles and providing supplemental coverage. States could pursue health-care reform through Medicare and Medicaid waivers.

Senator John Chafee of Rhode Island chaired the Senate Republican Health Care Task Force of a dozen-plus colleagues for more than three years. Their deliberations were introduced as *Health Equity Access Reform Today* (S.1770) on 22 November 1993. Reform of insurance markets would require guaranteed availability of coverage and community rating. Small employers and individuals could join purchasing cooperatives. Government subsidies for low-income individuals would be provided. A standard benefit package would be legislated by Congress. Medicare and Medicaid would be retained, although benefits would be cut. Tax treatment of health benefits would be limited.

Representative Jim Cooper of Tennessee, representing the conservative democratic forum, introduced the *Managed Competition Act of 1993* (H.R. 3222) on 6 October 1993. The bill would seek to reform purchasing incentives for consumers and provider financing and delivery incentives. A commission would specify a standard benefit package and pricing. Managed competition would utilize purchasing cooperatives and accountable health plans. Government subsidies would be available to low-income individuals. Employers would not be required to contribute to health insurance premiums and there would be limits on tax deductions. Medicare cuts would be pursued. Cost-containment is expected from competition, administrative savings, and malpractice reform. Medicare would remain, but Medicaid coverage would be phased into health alliances.

Representative Robert H. Michel, Republican of Illinois and the minority leader of the House introduced the *Affordable Health Care Now Act of 1993* (H.R. 3080) on 15 September 1993. This proposal would seek insurance reform and encourage group-purchasing agreements. Employers would be required to offer but not necessarily pay for health insurance for minimum benefits for their workers. Government subsidies would be offered to low-income individuals. The standard acute-care benefit package would be offered by cost-containment pursued through competition, administrative savings, and malpractice reform. Medicare—with higher premiums for high-income recipients—would remain, but Medicaid patients could be shifted to standard insurance plans by the states. This proposal advocates the least restructuring of the health-care enterprise.

While the legislative deliberations will no doubt end with a compromise featuring elements of the alternative proposals, they are certain to begin with the president's *Health Security Act*. The 1,342-page legislative draft reflects the concept of managed competition described above. The employer mandate for health insurance coverage was prominent in the work of the Pepper Commission. The proposal also attempts to address virtually every aspect of the health-care enterprise including initiatives in long-term care, rural communities, health research, academic health centers, public health, health personnel, antitrust reform, malpractice reform, workers' compensation, quality management, fraud and abuse, state responsibilities, and administrative simplification.

The details of restructuring financing of existing legislation, administrative modifications, and regulatory requirements is beyond the scope of this primer or perhaps any assessment short of a definitive analysis of health affairs at the threshold of the twenty-first century.

The Eilers-Angell criteria, or variations thereof, will challenge the deliberations on each of the proposals and their modification and amendment through the legislative debate. Subsequent struggles with implementation will focus on the role of federal and state governments, organization of purchasing mechanisms and delivery systems, and the allocation across society of the responsibility for financing health care.

Senator Russell Long, Democrat of Louisiana and Chairman of the Senate Finance Committee, was fond of saying, "Don't tax me. Don't tax thee. Tax that fellow behind the tree." Health policy is tax policy. And tax policy can contribute to expanding or containing health-care costs. The iron triangle of health care lurks in each of the proposals for health-care reform.

National health insurance seeks to address 260 million Americans. Now let us turn our attention to more modest demographic scales and consider the opportunities offered by the states respectively to pursue health-care reform.

Chapter 9
"To the States Respectively"

There are fifty natural laboratories
for health-care reform.

Health-care reform incorporates theories as yet untested in American society. Every health-policy action can have a reciprocal overreaction, and the more comprehensive and far-reaching the aspirations, the greater the potential for a major overreaction.[1] In health care, as in technology, small can be beautiful.

The fifty states—with populations ranging from about 500,000 in Wyoming and Vermont to 31 million in California, larger than the population of Canada—have in recent years been the central arenas of health-care reform. For certain purposes the states can collaborate, as Washington, Alaska, Montana, and Idaho (WAMI) do for medical education. The states represent manageable scale for health-care reform, and each is at lesser risk for a major overreaction. All but ten have populations smaller than that of Sweden, which a minister of health of India once described as an appropriate size for a demonstration project.

The Tenth Amendment of the Bill of Rights, reserving "to the states respectively" powers not given to the federal government or

101

prohibited to them, has guided the development of health policy for the last two centuries. The organization, financing, and delivery of health services have been predominantly a responsibility of the states. Among many other things, they regulate medical licensure, workers' compensation, health insurance, and hospital planning.

The first health department with a permanent board was established in Baltimore in 1793. Massachusetts founded the first state board of health in 1869. New York pioneered state legislation to regulate "the practice of physic and surgery" in 1797, and the Alabama legislature mandated regulation of the practice of dentistry in 1841.[2] Licensure of physicians, nurses, and other health professionals remains a state responsibility, and state initiatives have continued to guide health policy into the twentieth century. Wisconsin, in 1911, became the first state to pass legislation applying the principles of workers' compensation extensively. By 1935, comparable laws were adopted in half the states.[3]

Blue Cross and Blue Shield are regulated by the states, as are commercial insurance plans marketed nationwide. State regulation of market forces helped to launch certificate of need to control the expansion of hospitals and medical technology, much as public utilities control units of production.[4]

The Social Security Act of 1935 endorsed federal subsidization of state health programs through Title V (maternal and child health) and Title VI (public-health services). These matching and categorical grants are now found among a host of programs involved in the health-care system. A major expansion occurred in 1960 with the Kerr-Mills legislation subsidizing state programs for care of the aged, disabled, and indigent. Federal support increased even more dramatically in 1965 with Medicaid. In the 1980s, federal funding initiatives for state programs emphasized substance abuse and HIV. The states are suitable ground for attempting innovations—including the alternatives analyzed in the previous chapter—and for struggling with their implementation, learning from the experience, and transmitting the lessons for the whole society. This may be the strongest argument for expanding the role of the states beyond Medicaid, related health programs, and regulatory functions. What follow are discussions of a selected number of innovations adopted by individual states to finance and deliver health services.

Arizona

Although Medicaid was implemented in 1966 as a program of subsidy for health services at the state level, the Arizona legislature declined to enact the requisite participation until 1982, when the Arizona Health Care Cost-Containment System (AHCCCS) began operation as a Medicaid demonstration project.[5] By the end of its first year of operation, the program had served approximately 160,000 members. By 1990, enrollment had grown to more than 300,000. Nearly 9 percent of all adults and 20 percent of all children in the state have at one time or another been members of the system. Other states have observed this experiment to see what can be learned.

The principal goal of the Arizona system was to deliver an alternative health program to the poor that would be more cost-effective than conventional Medicaid programs. As a demonstration project, the Arizona system obtained a waiver to exempt it from providing many services mandated in other Medicaid programs, including long-term care, family planning, mental-health care, and a number of services for children. The provision of health services to indigent populations became the responsibility of counties through contracts with private groups. Cost-containment measures included minimal copayments for visits to physicians and for prescription medication.

The key element of the cost-containment strategy, however, was replacing the fee-for-service reimbursement mechanism of traditional Medicaid plans with a capitated payment. The Arizona system derives its funding from three sources: federal, state, and county dollars. A capitation rate has been determined for each eligibility category. Federal matching funds are provided for approximately 62 percent of the appropriate capitation rate multiplied by the estimated number of Arizonans in the program, with quarterly adjustments for actual enrollment. The funding mechanism places the responsibility for controlling health-care expenditures on state government.

Health services under AHCCCS are provided by prepaid health plans, which are awarded contracts through competitive bidding. Enrollment in one of the thirteen participating plans is mandatory for all members. Because the state reimburses the contracted provider on a capitated basis, the plan accepts the risk for keeping down costs.

The Arizona system has not gone without criticism.[6] It has inadequately addressed the 500,000 Arizonans without health insurance. One applicant out of every four reports that the AHCCCS application process is very difficult. To address the problem of the uninsured, Arizona launched a project to establish a health plan for employees of small businesses, and it now struggles with the challenge to extend the program to rural areas. It is hoped that AHCCCS will become self-sufficient in the 1990s.

Hawaii

Hawaii is a natural demonstration project in health affairs. Its many islands, with a land area of 6,400 square miles, are home to approximately 1.2 million inhabitants, a third of them Caucasian, a fifth people of Japanese descent, and the remainder of Hawaiian, Filipino, Chinese, and other ancestry. The population of Hawaii is younger on average than that of the other states, with proportionally fewer people sixty-five and older. Approximately 320,000 military personnel, their families, and retirees are eligible for medical care by Tripler Army Hospital, effectively reducing the size of the population dependent on the Hawaiian health plan. These demographics naturally influence the morbidity experience and health-care needs of the state.

More than three-quarters of Hawaii's residents live on the island of Oahu, in and around the city of Honolulu. Hawaii's economy focuses on tourism, agriculture, and the military, and the state has enjoyed remarkable economic growth. The state is distinguished in several respects. It has 3.1 general hospital beds per thousand population—as compared with an average of 4.5 for the nation as a whole. The physician-to-population ratio is higher than on the mainland. Approximately one-third of physicians practice in multispecialty groups, three times the national average. Blue Cross, Blue Shield, the Straub Clinic, and the Kaiser Permanente are the principal competitors for subscribers.

The Hawaii Prepaid Health Plan Act of 1974 requires employers to provide coverage meeting established standards.[7] It has resulted in an expansion of coverage in terms of both population and comprehensiveness of benefits. Added to Medicare, Medicaid, and existing third-party health insurance, the plan has given Hawaii universal health insurance since 1980. Employers must provide health-insurance coverage for all full-time employees—those working twenty hours or more a week—and pay at least half the premium cost of the coverage. Payment for employees' dependents is not required. The choice for employers has been to promote universal coverage or pay increased taxes to expand Medicaid.

The competition in Hawaii gives the universal health insurance administered by private plans a greater probability of success, as does the remarkably low hospital utilization—360 bed days per thousand enrollees. The pattern of development in Hawaii was established many years ago with payment for outpatient care as a typical mode of insurance; by contrast, most health insurance focuses almost exclusively on inpatient hospitalization. Hawaii's health-insurance plan was influenced by group-practice physicians who favored a combination of hospital and medical-service coverage over the distinction emphasized by Medicare Parts A and B, which mimic Blue Cross and Blue Shield.

The Hawaiian plan has been successful in expanding coverage, but it has flaws. Some small businesses in Hawaii have dropped their life-insurance benefits in order to keep offering the state-mandated health benefits to their employees. The Hawaiian system may not be workable for the nation as a whole. If individual states mandate that employers insure workers, businesses may move to bordering states, as a number of Massachusetts businesses did. That alternative, of course, is not available in Hawaii. Less than 2 percent of the total population of Hawaii has no coverage. Medicare addresses 7 percent, Medicaid 11 percent, the Civilian Health and Medical Program of the United States (CHAMPUS) 27 percent, and private insurance 53 percent.[8]

Indiana

As Indiana experienced a rapid increase in the size and frequency of medical malpractice claims in the 1970s, availability of insurance for hospitals and physicians decreased dramatically. Governor Otis R. Bowen, a physician, called for reform of the tort system for medical malpractice in 1975, and the Indiana General Assembly responded quickly, enacting the Medical Malpractice Act. The reforms

thereby legislated were among the first comprehensive medical malpractice reforms in the nation. They have undergone few significant
changes since.

The purpose of the Indiana Medical Malpractice Act was never
specifically stated by the legislature. The Indiana Supreme Court,
however, found that the act was passed to protect the public from
decreased medical services when health-care providers limited their
practices owing to cancelation of malpractice coverage.[9]

The act contains many major reforms. First, total damages recover-
able for any one injury may not exceed $750,000. Second, no claim
may be brought against a health-care provider unless it has been filed
within two years of the alleged occurrence; an exception is made for
minors under six, who have until age eighteen to file actions. Third,
malpractice plaintiffs must file their claims with the state insurance
department's medical review panel—an attorney, as nonvoting chair,
and three health-care providers—before proceeding to trial. The panel
provides expert opinion on the cause of the injury and the liability of
the defendant but plays no role in determining damages. The opinion
of the panel is admissible at trial, but it is not conclusive evidence of
liability. The panel members may be called to testify by either party.

Plaintiffs also have the option of bypassing the medical review
panel if all parties consent, and they can opt out unilaterally if their
claims are under $15,000. The parties can settle a claim at any time. A
plaintiffs' compensation fund may evaluate and pay any claim without
the guidance of a panel opinion; a state-run insurance fund pays large
claims. A health-care provider who qualifies under the statute is liable
only up to $100,000 for an occurrence of malpractice. When a court
issues a verdict for more than $100,000, the excess, up to the damage
limit, is paid by the plaintiffs' compensation fund.

Three other key reforms include the formation of the Residual
Malpractice Insurance Authority, an organization that provides primary malpractice insurance for physicians who are unable to obtain
coverage; the requirement that the insurance commissioner report
judgments against health-care professionals to their licensure boards;
and the limiting of attorney fees to a maximum of 15 percent of any
recovery from the fund.

Approximately 90 percent of Indiana hospitals and almost all Indiana physicians participate in the state plan. If a health-care provider fails to meet the prerequisites of the act, the malpractice plaintiff will not be restricted by its terms.

The reforms instituted in Indiana have been extremely successful in reducing the malpractice premiums paid by health-care professionals. Indiana health-care providers pay among the lowest premiums in the nation, and providers and insurers are satisfied with the system. Critics point to the delays associated with the medical review panels. Nevertheless, one analyst notes that both the medical profession and the insurance industry regard Indiana as providing a model for successful reduction of malpractice claims. Tort reform for malpractice liability is high on the agenda for most practicing physicians, and the other forty-nine states can study and learn from Indiana's bold steps.[10]

Iowa

Land-grant colleges and universities supported across the country by the Morrill Act of 1862 have linked education and research to the community through extension services.[11] College-level educational programs in agronomy, soil sciences, and other disciplines have extended their influence not only in the preparation of graduates for the state but also in the organization of research units and model farms.

The University of Iowa, a land-grant institution in Iowa City, has one of the largest referral medical centers in the nation, with 900 beds, almost 200 clinics, and a staff of 7,000, including 1,200 physicians and 1,500 nurses.[12] It is the regional hub for the 120 hospitals in Iowa, which serve some 100 counties and 3 million residents. The University of Iowa Hospital and Clinics, with its affiliated schools of medicine and nursing, has educated most of the physicians, nurses, and hospital administrators in these institutions. It provides continuing-education programs and conducts biomedical and health-services research to enhance patient care, in addition to serving as a referral base for specialized and technologically sophisticated services, often at the stage of clinical trials. The academic health center in Iowa City serves as a nucleus of a regional system. Patients come to the center on referral from physicians practicing in the 100 community hospitals of 150 beds or less and the almost two dozen regional hospitals of up to 650 beds.

Reciprocally, graduates from the College of Medicine and the residency and fellowship programs sponsored by the University Hospital and Clinics fan out through the state and beyond. Advances in biomedical research are widely disseminated, and specialty consultation is readily available.

The University of Iowa was the prototype for the regionalizing of health services that came about with the legislation of regional medical programs in 1965, an effort to bring the nation's more than 100 academic health centers and affiliated hospitals together with medical practitioners, community hospitals, and other health resources.[13] As the regional referral center for hospitals throughout the state, the University of Iowa Hospital and Clinics is also a prototype for a publicly supported health-care system. It approximates the model of the "coordinated health-service areas" on which the Hill-Burton legislation of 1946 was based. The Iowa model is not easily replicated, however, as many states lack a single or dominant tertiary medical center. In my own state of Pennsylvania, seven academic health centers compete for patients and resources.

Maryland

In 1971, the Maryland General Assembly established the Health Services Cost Review Commission (HSCRC) as an independent body within the Department of Health and Mental Hygiene.[14] Charged with curbing increases in costs and charges, the HSCRC had responsibility for ensuring that total costs were reasonably related to the services provided, that rates charged were reasonably related to costs incurred, that rates charged patients or groups of patients were equitable, and that no undue discrimination was practiced in the establishment of hospital rates. Using a variety of methods, the commission set prospective rates. These methods included comparing one hospital's costs to those of another, limiting the size of hospital rate increases, and denying high-cost hospitals any increases. Since 1974, hospitals have been required to charge commission-approved rates. The system has successfully controlled costs and charges within Maryland hospitals.

In developing its rate-setting procedures, the cost commission outlined five operating principles: cost control rather than profit control, resource use rather than payment control, budget constraints rather than managerial preemption, advanced establishment of attainable performance parameters rather than arbitrary targets, and medical practice and trustee responsibility rather than physician-controlled hospital care. One trade-off is recognized within the state's system. Payers who pay on discharge or within thirty days receive a 2 percent discount, and those allowing open enrollment or group conversion in their health-benefit plans receive a 4 percent discount. These discounts encourage prompt payment and group-rate insurance. They are also designed to offset the allocation of uncompensated care, estimated at approximately 4 percent of total inpatient care. The commission reviews hospital costs quarterly to ensure that hospitals are receiving reimbursement for their costs. Inflation adjustments, discounts for Medicare and Medicaid, discounts for prompt payment, and volume adjustments to reflect true variable cost allocation are used.

With a population of 4.5 million and sixty general hospitals, Maryland has implemented a regulatory mechanism for hospital cost controls. It is one of fewer than a dozen states to attempt such regulation. But for Maryland, complications notwithstanding, it works.[15]

Massachusetts

The Scots Charitable Society of Boston was organized in 1657 to help the sick, aid the poor, and bury the dead. This initiative was followed in 1662 by creation of the first almshouse in the colonies for care of the indigent. Three centuries later, legislation was proposed mandating third-party health-insurance coverage to be paid by employers. At the time, the state was basking in the so-called Massachusetts miracle of high employment and expanding tax coffers. Health policy became tax policy in Massachusetts.

The plan was intended to provide coverage for uninsured workers, the unemployed, disabled children and adults, and college students lacking health insurance. It was pursued as mandatory employer coverage, or a "compulsory contribution," but it entailed tax subsidies both directly and indirectly, overtly and covertly, in the form of redistribution of income.

The plan made Massachusetts the first state after Hawaii to legislate mandated health care. The Massachusetts Health Security Act, signed by Governor Michael Dukakis in 1988, represented a play-or-pay approach in that it did not technically require employers to provide health insurance; rather it made companies with more than five employees pay a penalty of $1,680 per employee if they failed to offer coverage. One factor that facilitated passage of the Massachusetts plan was the state's budget surplus and its low unemployment rate—about half the national average. This healthy economic climate made possible the financial commitment to cover those left out of employer plans, such as unemployed people ineligible for Medicaid. The state's relatively generous Medicaid program left a manageable group of poor people to add to the state's financial responsibility. States with larger numbers of poor uninsured residents would have to pay much more.

The plan sought universal coverage. Implementation, however, has been deferred until 1995. Many observers cite a fiscal crisis and the election of a conservative governor on the issues of state finance for the difficulties. Others note the slim majority by which the legislation passed and emphasize a lack of political conviction and of feasibility of implementation.[16] Like Medicare a quarter of a century before, the plan sought access without restructuring of health services in an environment of the highest health-care costs in the country. A comparison of Massachusetts and Hawaii provides a dramatic case-analysis of the multiplicity of factors that shape the implementation of health-care reform.

Minnesota

The Twin Cities of Minneapolis and St. Paul had thirty-three hospitals in 1984. Four years later, eight hospitals had closed, and others had consolidated into three hospital systems with four teaching and two independent hospitals remaining. The dynamic changes began in 1973 when St. Louis Park Medical Center developed a provider-based insurance organization. This group hoped to provide an alternative to Blue Cross and Blue Shield as a third-party intermediary, channeling money directly for medical care. Interactions with satellite groups created a network of primary-care and specialty physicians. The success of such organizations alarmed the county medical societies, causing them to create their own provider groups. Combining physician groups also meant combining the facilities they used, and the first wave of hospital closings began. Unprofitable facilities merged or went under. The end result is the existence of networks of physicians, hospitals, and clinics.

Much like the consolidated hospitals, HMOs joined to form some of the nation's largest health-care-delivery systems. In 1991, two HMOs with a total of 650,000 enrollees merged. In an effort to reduce total health-care expenditures by at least 10 percent, a coalition of corporations (Business Health Care Action Group [BHCAG]) contracted with a consortium of providers to deliver services to their employees. The employer coalition boasted fourteen major Twin Cities corporations, including Dayton Hudson and Pillsbury. The resultant combination of services and facilities shifted the delivery of health care in the Twin Cities to community-based managed-care services and implemented the prototypes of health alliances and accountable health plans advocated in health-care reform.

The dynamic flux of health-care restructuring continues in Minneapolis–St. Paul. The arrival of 1994 saw five major players—Allina, Health Partners, Fairview System, Health East, and Minnesota Health System—dominating the market. The development of five integrated network systems from thirty-three hospitals with their respective medical staffs in less than a decade represents dramatic health-care restructuring. It also suggests that the end may not be in sight. It is important to recognize that this ferment is taking place in a single metropolitan area with a population of approximately 2.6 million, one-hundredth of the population for which we seek health-care reform.[17]

The uninsured—without an advocate in most states—have not been forgotten in Minnesota. In 1992, Governor Arnie Carlson signed a law enacting HealthRight (now called MinnesotaCare), a program addressed to reducing overall costs and providing care for those unable to get it through current payment strategies. Funds will come from a variety of sources, including an additional five-cent tax on cigarettes, a 2 percent tax on gross revenues of providers (hospitals and physicians), and a 1 percent tax on the gross premiums of nonprofit health insurance. The participation of physicians is ensured, as those who decline to accept MinnesotaCare patients are disqualified from treating Medicare, Medicaid, and workers' compensation patients, as well as state employees. Other goals of the plan include eliminating risk ratings, establishing practice guidelines, and increasing by 20 percent the number of primary-care physicians in the state.

The Minneapolis–St. Paul experience can be likened to that of Rochester, New York, where Eastman Kodak and Xerox, like *Fortune* 500 companies in Minnesota, have had a major influence on health-care reform. In Rochester, though, the companies work through Blue Cross and Blue Shield, which control 80 percent of the market. The private and independent sectors are collaborating to use incentives and constraints to move health care toward cost-effective services. These bottom-up approaches test the problem-solving skills of health-care providers.

New Jersey

New Jersey launched an all-payer system for hospital care in the early 1980s. The goal was to create a standardized per-case payment system to eliminate cost shifting among payers and provide an assessment for uncompensated service so inner-city hospitals could survive and patients would not be denied care. Policy makers and health analysts alike watched to see the results of instituting a prospective-payment model based on diagnostic-related groups developed at Yale University.

The roots of New Jersey's involvement with hospital rate regulation go back three decades. In 1961, the state placed a cap on Blue Cross per diem reimbursement. A decade later, a voluntary budget-review program was initiated under the administration of the New Jersey Hospital Association. During its tenure from 1971 to 1974, the program had no significant impact on health costs. In 1975, the state moved to a more rigorous cost-containment strategy with the implementation of the Standard Hospital Accounting and Rate Evaluation. Per diem rates were set for Blue Cross and Medicaid, whose combined reimbursement accounted for half of hospital inpatient revenues. The program demonstrated a statistically significant reduction in the annual increase in hospital expenditures per adjusted patient day during 1977 and 1978.[18]

In 1978, the New Jersey legislature enacted Chapter 83, a law creating a payment system designed to force hospitals to make more efficient use of resources. Proponents argued that the all-payer regulation at the heart of the bill would eliminate cost shifting to nonregulated payers. The law also attempted to alleviate the financial difficulties of hospitals with high numbers of indigent patients and to improve hospital access for the uninsured. To these ends it sought to ensure that universal hospital rate regulation encompassed all payers, that the reimbursement system reflected case-mix variations among hospitals, that all payers shared responsibility for uncompensated care, and that hospitals received an infusion of working capital. Although Chapter 83 is often called the DRG law, the act stipulated only that reimbursement take into account case-mix variation; the choice of payment mechanisms was left to the New Jersey Department of Health. Implementation of the plan began in 1980, and by 1982 all hospitals in the state had been enrolled.

What has been the effect of New Jersey's all-payer system? Supporters argue that the system controls costs: New Jersey's cost per adjusted admission was $3,774 in 1988, considerably less than the $4,629 average for hospitals in the Northeast. It is also true that the DRG system has resulted in lower costs per admission. Under the all-payer system, however, the state has experienced an increase in admissions that largely offsets the savings, so that the overall effect of DRGs in controlling costs has been negligible.

The New Jersey system has been facing mounting criticism in recent years. One point of contention has been the program's method of financing uncompensated care. The DRG rates include a markup to cover the cost of charity care and bad debts. The surcharge monies are placed in a trust fund that pays hospital bills for selected New Jersey residents. In 1992, a district court handed down a decision rendering the method of collection for the fund illegal. The judge decided in favor of labor unions that sued the New Jersey Hospital Association, claiming exemption from the surcharges on their self-funded health-insurance plans as protected under the Employee Retirement Income Security Act (ERISA).[19] The Court of Appeals for the Third Circuit reversed and remanded the decision; the unions have appealed to the Supreme Court. As other states, too, take the lead in health policy, it is likely there will be further legal challenges.

Oregon

The debate over setting health-care priorities in Oregon began in 1988 when state lawmakers decided to eliminate Medicaid funding for organ transplants and to increase coverage for pregnant women instead. The highly publicized death from leukemia of a seven-year-old boy named Coby Howard, who might have lived had he received a bone-marrow transplant, forced an emotional and difficult debate.[20] The critical policy issue was the equity of providing sophisticated and costly services to a few Oregonians covered under Medicaid before providing basic services to other needy citizens, including the working poor who lacked any public or private coverage.

The Oregon health-care plan emerged in the wake of the turmoil over the transplant decision. In 1989, a commission of five physicians, a public-health nurse, a social worker, and four consumers was created to solicit public involvement through community meetings aimed at building a consensus on the values that would guide resource allocation. This experiment has claimed national attention. The field of medical ethics has, in effect, moved from university seminars and symposia to the political arena.

A strong component of the Oregon plan is its facing up to limited resources. It is not being touted as a cost-containment policy. At the time of its proposal, Dr. John Kitzhaber, the president of the state senate, publicly claimed that the state did not anticipate saving much money but rather viewed the program as a means for the public and for policy makers to make informed decisions.

The definitions of "basic health services" could tie up a graduate-level seminar for an entire semester. Most analysts acknowledge the likelihood of the continued existence of a tiered system.[21] I liken this to the first class / business class / tourist system of air travel. It is very appealing until you try to allocate services. If "tourist" represents the public good, we all agree on prenatal care, immunization, and the repair of a cleft lip and palate in a newborn as qualifying needs. Cosmetic surgery, on the other hand, is readily allocated to first class. But where do we put the vast majority of health services, which are not directed at life-threatening conditions and which in fact contribute little to health status but do much to ameliorate "dis-ease"? The citizens of Oregon, under the leadership of John Kitzhaber, were willing to make the difficult judgments.[22]

First estimates, published in May 1990, were based on an evaluation of 1,600 disorders. A revision announced in February 1991 was based on 800 disorders. Pneumonia, tuberculosis, peritonitis, appendicitis, and hernia with obstruction topped the list. Kidney cysts, terminal AIDS, chronic pancreatitis, and extremely low birth weight earned the lowest priority.

Advocates of the Oregon plan emphasize the major advantage it has over the current program: it brings uninsured Oregonians into the health-care system. The Oregon plan directly confronts the fact that the United States is not going to provide every conceivable medical service to everyone, especially not through its public programs. The plan inspires fierce opposition, however. It explicitly condones the withholding of care, a practice widely viewed as unacceptable in the United States, where a physician or hospital accepting a patient for treatment, even one who is uninsured, is morally and legally bound to provide the necessary medical care, and the reimbursement and service decisions are somewhat separated. In the Oregon proposal, they are joined, and the law sanctions withholding some medically beneficial services.

The ideas advocated in Oregon will most likely be pursued differently in the independent sector and probably not at all in the private sector. Without public-sector support or third-party coverage, however, few if any of us could afford sophisticated biomedical treatments. The initiatives in Oregon will help the rest of the country identify and debate the alternatives for resource allocation.

Washington

The state just to the north of Oregon is not to be outdone in the arena of health-care reform. Its Health Services Act of 1993 is meant to blend market incentives and regulation in order to provide access to health care for everyone.[23] It specifies seven objectives: (1) to create a reformed system that uses private providers and facilities to allow consumers to choose among competing plans operating within budget limits and regulations that promote the public good; (2)

to enroll state residents in certified health plans of their choice that meet state standards regarding affordability, accessibility, cost-effectiveness, and clinical efficacy; (3) to permit state residents to choose from a full range of health-care providers with good health-services management, quality assurance, and cost-effectiveness; (4) to involve all state residents, businesses, employees, and government in payment for health services, with total cost to individuals on a sliding scale based on income; (5) to give individuals and businesses the option to purchase any health services they may choose in addition to those contained in the uniform benefits package; (6) to coordinate the delivery, purchase, and provision of health services among the federal, state, and local governments; and (7) to keep the rate of increase in the total cost of health services similar to the rate of personal-income growth within a publicly regulated private marketplace that preserves personal choice. These objectives are consistent with those of the Clinton reform program.

The act envisions phased implementation over a six-year period, beginning with enrollment expansion for the basic health plan that has been operative since 1987.[24] Other initial steps include the creation of a commission composed of five persons appointed by the governor and charged with developing the uniform benefits package within strict cost limitations. This package will include all the services offered by the basic health plan, as well as pharmacy services, reproductive services, preventive dentistry for children, and some mental-health and chemical-dependency treatment.

In January 1995 the commission is to submit to the legislature a proposed uniform benefits package, analyses of the economic impact on small businesses and on low-income families, and certification standards for health plans. The uniform benefits package will be offered through certified health plans in July 1995. The HMO and other service contracts are to become effective January 1996.

Medical coverage cannot be denied to individuals because of preexisting conditions; preventive services will be encouraged. A health-insurance purchasing cooperative will seek to pool risk and provide coverage. First-year implementation also includes liability reform and imposition of tobacco, liquor, and hospital taxes.

Phasing of coverage begins in 1994 with expansion of Medicaid to children living at up to 200 percent of the federal poverty level. Employers with 500 or more employees must provide coverage by July 1995 and must include dependents by July 1996. At that time, employers with 100 or more employees will have to provide coverage, followed by coverage for dependents the next year, when employers with fewer than 100 employees will have to begin providing coverage.

The state of Washington, with a population of 5 million, has undertaken an ambitious program of reform. Given its complexity, the plan will doubtless face a number of difficulties. Dealing as it does, however, with a population only 2 percent the size of the entire United States population, it appears to be working on a manageable scale.

Two decades after the British enacted the National Health Service, Medicare launched national health insurance for the elderly in American society. One decade later, Hawaii pioneered the state version of national health insurance. Now health-care reform is a lead issue on state as well as federal agendas: three-quarters of the states have implemented, legislated, or drafted reform measures.

A federal-state partnership enjoys priority in political rhetoric but is ever elusive in implementation. Forging such a partnership will involve issues more complex than those involved in tax policy alone, but an effective collaboration will be needed to address as formidable a human-service need as that for health care. The federal government represents expertise, resources, and a national scope of concern; the states are better equipped to bring health, education, and welfare programs together in their own communities. The next chapter discusses the common mission of federal and state agencies: promotion of the general welfare.

Chapter 10
Promoting the General Welfare

Societal entitlements are relative,
not absolute.

Two centuries after the Declaration of Independence proclaimed that all people "are endowed by their Creator with certain unalienable rights," Americans struggle to ensure rights that they view not as guaranteed by a supernatural power but as achieved through societal entitlements. One person's right or benefit, moreover, is often realized at another person's cost.

Are there "unalienable rights" to health or health care? If not, are Americans ready to declare a societal entitlement comparable to the one declared for the elderly in 1965? Efforts to answer these questions require greater understanding of the society's capacity to meet health-care needs for individuals and for the population at large.

Although the Bill of Rights articulates several of the unalienable rights in American society—including security against unreasonable search and seizure, the right to a speedy, fair trial and an impartial jury, the right to counsel—it nowhere guarantees health care. Nor, for that matter, does it guarantee education. For me, both are rights implied in the Constitution's aim to "promote the general welfare." That requires access to health care as well as to an education. American society recognized the latter need a century and a half ago; it is time to acknowledge the need for access to health care. Education, of course, is a societal entitlement rather than an unalienable right. Government, religious institutions, and independent schools make the entitlement a reality. The society is now enjoined to create a similar entitlement for health care.

I ask my students, "Do we have a right to health care in our society?" The answer is almost unanimously "No." Several of the more astute students suggest that the elderly have an entitlement in Medicare. Then I ask, "Do we have a right to an education in the United State?" They respond, "Yes." Then I ask if the educational entitlement includes a Ph.D. at M.I.T. "Of course not" is their reply. Next I ask if the quality of elementary and secondary education is comparable across geographic and political jurisdictions. "Of course not," they say.

In offering a public education through grade twelve financed by tax dollars, the society recognizes that entitlement may imply relative equity and quality. The public education available in the wealthy suburbs of some major cities has advantages over that offered in many inner-city schools. Affluence also provides some students with the benefit of books, pocket calculators, and personal computers and with the advantages that may be provided by parochial or independent schools. Similarly, the health status of the affluent reflects advantages in housing, nutrition, recreation, personal security, and other aspects of lifestyle.

The right to public education was enacted by the legislature of the Commonwealth of Massachusetts in 1848.[1] One can assume that the legislators saw evidence that an education was beneficial to society as well as to individuals. Evidence for the benefits of health care other than in the areas of sanitation and control of epidemics would not be perceived until well into the twentieth century. A healthy population was always desirable, but there seemed to be few measures that could be undertaken to make a difference.

In the final decade of the twentieth century there are abundant measures. Paradoxically, we can do more to make a difference for any given individual than we can afford to do for all individuals in the population. The issue of health-care entitlement must address the needs of both the population and the individual in the context of finite resources.

Absolute Aspiration and Variable Entitlement

The right to health care exercised by one citizen can diminish the availability of care for another. Resources—especially biomedical technology, health personnel, and hospitals—given over to renal dialysis or a coronary artery bypass graft for one citizen are not available to a patient waiting for a liver transplant or, for that matter, to a classroom of children in need of polio vaccine. Equity in the pursuit of health care as a right requires resource allocation. Choices—who, what, how much, and when—are inevitable.

In 1948 the British National Health Service established health care as both an absolute and a relative right. Each citizen had the right to register with a general practitioner for all primary care. The frequency, duration, and quality of their encounters varied. Secondary and tertiary care were provided on referral by the general practitioner to hospital-based consultants, who controlled access to their services through waiting lists. The patient waited for elective surgery, such as treatment of hemorrhoids, repair of hernias, tonsillectomies, hysterectomies, and, more recently, total hip replacements and other technologically sophisticated procedures. The wait for a relatively minor, nonurgent procedure, such as a hernia repair, could last for years in some regions of the country. Such a delay would be construed as a denial of health care in the United States, not as part of a right. Moreover, the British physician controlled the allocation of that right.

In the Canadian system inaugurated two decades later, the right was once again both absolute and relative. The current program is comprehensive in intent. Both the federal and the provincial governments attempt to deliver on the right by adopting resource allocation to meet patient needs. Fee schedules for physicians and global budgeting for hospitals provide Canadians with an opportunity for health care but impose constraints on the realization of their right to it. As in the United Kingdom, allocation decisions are delegated to the physician after public officials determine the budget.

Because health services can mean the difference between life and death, we feel compelled to view them in absolute terms. America's insistence on absolutes in health care has inhibited its ability to guarantee access to basic health services for every individual. Access, quality, and cost containment cannot be achieved in absolute terms. Access to basic health services for all Americans, like access to elementary and secondary education, can be provided only as a relative right. Further, a definition of basic health services is not as clear as a definition of the basic educational rights. By beginning with health promotion, preventive services, and primary care, however, one can build a concept of affordable health services.

Like the United Kingdom and Canada, the United States has had to make compromises in the distribution of health care. In the United Kingdom there is de jure rationing of health care. In the United States health-care rationing is de facto. The Canadian system combines aspects of both approaches. The United Kingdom gives priority to equity. The United States gives priority to excellence. Canada searches for a balance. American society, while proclaiming the finest health care in the world, offers excellence for the fortunate at the expense of access for all. Current public discourse and political debate would suggest that "we the people" wish to modify that equation in order to "promote the general welfare." One hears public officials, labor leaders, corporate executives, and—increasingly—physicians declare, "Health care is a right."

Entitlements in American society appear to be relative rather than absolute. Every American is entitled, for example, to equal protection under the law, but the ability to afford costly legal counsel enhances that entitlement; lack of such resources tends to diminish it. An American, on reaching age sixty-five, is entitled to Social Security benefits. The size of the monthly check, however, can reflect the amount of social insurance paid by the individual during his or her working years.

For most of the population sixty-five or older, access to health care approaches that of the universal system in Canada and, in some instances, exceeds it. Total hip replacement, coronary artery bypass graft surgery, and chronic renal dialysis are available in the United States for the elderly virtually on demand. Medicare beneficiaries have the right to physician services paid for under Part B and to hospitalization within certain limits under Part A. Medicare payment schedules, deductibles, limited Medigap insurance coverage, and balance billing by the physician, taken together, curtail the scope of that right. The elderly have a right to only limited extended care in nursing homes but enjoy extensive services for terminal illness through hospice care. Long-term nursing care, except where provided through Medicaid when the individual or family has drained all financial resources, is not an entitlement. The elderly in our society, however, have a right to health care that equals or surpasses, both quantitatively and qualitatively, the rights of the young to an education.

Medicaid is not guaranteed by the federal government; it is a state prerogative that draws on a federal subsidy. The disparities of this right are illustrated by the contrasts between the most generous programs—those in California and New York—and those in Mississippi and West Virginia, where a bare minimum is provided. In the wealthier states the federal government subsidizes 50 percent of the costs, while in the poorer states, 79 percent of the costs are subsidized.[2]

Veterans of the American armed forces are entitled to hospital and medical care through the Department of Medicine and Surgery of the Veterans Administration. Approximately 23 million veterans are beneficiaries.[3] As federal beneficiaries, Native Americans living on reservations enjoy health care as a right. The Indian Health Service on the Navajo reservation resembles the British National Health Service in terms of regionalization of services, resource allocation, and centralized budgeting. The program attempts to go beyond anything available through the public sector to immigrants and the descendants of immigrants.

Corporate America makes a formidable contribution to providing tens of millions of people with an entitlement to health care. The beneficiaries, of course, are limited mainly to those employed by or retired from large corporations. Third-party coverage through Blue Cross, Blue Shield, commercial insurance companies, or HMOs is provided as a fringe benefit. For some employees and their families, the benefit is as generous as any in the United Kingdom or Canada.

For the two-thirds of the population that enjoys something close to entitlement to the finest health care in the world, the society does indeed "promote the general welfare." The vulnerability of this entitlement, however, is being demonstrated by layoffs, revisions of benefits, and cancellation of coverage. For almost 40 million Americans, however, health care is at best a charity granted by various institutions and providers. These individuals lack third-party health-insurance coverage, are too young for Medicare, and have incomes above the level at which they would be eligible for Medicaid in most states. They are not necessarily without all medical care, however; often they benefit from the charitable and voluntary services of hospitals and physicians. Paradoxically, although secondary and tertiary care is available, primary care and preventive medicine are not. Some form of cross-subsidization is called for; health professionals, technology, and facilities must be paid for somehow. And one person's cross-subsidization is another's cost shifting.

Financial Coverage

Health-care financing can be evaluated in terms of the following life stages: the initial years (birth to age twenty), the working years (twenties into the sixties), and the retirement years (sixties, seventies, and—increasingly—eighties and nineties). These categories do not represent discrete segments of the population; there is overlap. Some individuals join the workforce at sixteen or younger, while others, such as many professionals, do not embark on independent careers until their thirties. At the other end of the spectrum, while some professionals fight retirement at age sixty-five, and indeed continue to work into their seventies and eighties, others are delighted with the thought of early retirement. Nonetheless, one can speak of the median experience of these groups. The health care of each has been addressed by health and social policy in different ways.

The modern era of federal health policy began in 1935 with a categorical approach for determining beneficiaries. The categorical strategy persists sixty years later. Whether or not universal access to a basic package of health benefits is enacted by the 103rd or a subsequent Congress, there is merit in thinking about the population in broad age categories with differing, albeit overlapping, needs. For the initial decades, we should envision universal access and innovative systems linking health, education, and social services; for the working years, health benefits for employees of small businesses, portability of benefits between jobs, and health benefits for the unemployed; and for the retirement years, coverage for long-term care and medical prescriptions. These initiatives are certainly not exhaustive, but they clearly indicate a credible priority.

Thinking of, and referring to, national health insurance as a single concept restricts our adaptive imagination and creativity. A flexible tripartite strategy could offer viable opportunities for raising resources in a pragmatic, equitable fashion that is comprehensible to the employer, the worker, and the individual voter. Federal guidelines for matching funds through Medicaid waivers to the states could encourage innovative strategies focused on population groups. Project grants for development of health-care systems and for purchase of services could promote cost-effectiveness as well as equity and quality in the organization and delivery of health services. While such an approach lacks the clarity, simplicity, or comprehensiveness of the Canadian and British systems, it is consistent with the American experience of pragmatism, pluralism, and incrementalism.

THE INITIAL DECADES

Over the past quarter-century the federal government has made expenditures in excess of one trillion dollars on behalf of those sixty-five years and older. The rationale at the time of Medicare's enactment was an endorsement of social principles that can be traced back to Bismarck in Germany in the late 1800s. In the 1990s the average white female reaching age sixty-five can expect to live another two decades. If health care is guaranteed in the last two decades of life, why not in the first two as well? Such a commitment would be an investment in the nation's future, which is certainly as important as its past. The time has come for building on initiatives already taken on behalf of infants, children, and youth.

The principal health problems in the first two decades of life are teenage pregnancy, premature births, infant mortality, congenital malformations, and mental and physical handicaps. Each of these problems requires a spectrum of human services that range far beyond medical care and the ministrations of physicians. Whereas Medicare implemented three-decade-old concepts, a strategy adequate to the needs of infants, children, and adolescents, including pregnant teenagers, must synthesize medical care, education, social services, and public health. Almost two decades ago, "Kiddie Care," patterned after Medicare, was advocated; I would argue that restructuring and innovation of services must accompany financing.

In 1963 and 1965, amendments to Title V of the Social Security Act created grants-in-aid to cover 75 percent of the costs of comprehensive health services for infants, children, and youth in certain population groups. State and local health departments, schools of medicine, and affiliated teaching hospitals became the providers. The legislation required that a project coordinate services with state or local health, education, and welfare programs and include at least "screening, diagnosis, preventive services, treatment, correction of defects, and aftercare, both medical and dental."

The Child Health Act of 1967 extended the programs for five years and added authorization for payment of reasonable costs of inpatient hospital services. An amendment aimed at cost-effectiveness called for maximum use of health personnel with varying levels of training. Accordingly, new personnel with knowledge of the social, cultural, and demographic structure of the population complemented and supplemented the efforts of traditional health professionals. This legislation built on the past and forecast the future.

A program of early and periodic screening, diagnosis, and treatment (EPSDT) represents yet another incremental initiative in pursuit of comprehensive health services for infants and children. The Women's and Infant Care Program (WIC) for subsidizing nutritional supplements recognizes that the achievement of health requires more than simply medical care.[4] These initiatives were built incrementally to elaborate services in a cumulative fashion. Unfortunately, they related more closely to the welfare paradigm of means-tested eligibility than to the entitlement represented by education.

Head Start offers a prototype.[5] For a generation, preschoolers in

Head Start have benefited from a coordinated group of health, education, and social-welfare programs. Many professionals concerned with policy consider it the most successful of the Great Society's efforts.

Plans for national health insurance for mothers, pregnant women, infants, children, and adolescents should draw on community-based models. Providing immunization, preventing accidents, and dealing with the problems of teenage pregnancy and adolescent drug abuse require a coordinated medical, educational, and welfare approach. Close collaboration between and among schools, public-health agencies, and health-care systems is essential in a proactive strategy. Families should have the prerogative of using alternative health-care plans—the equivalents, in education, of parochial and independent schools. Although many families choose such schools over public ones, the importance of public education and the legitimate obligations of the taxpayer persist.

I propose that we begin health-care reform at the base of the demographic profile. The goal is to use innovative health-care systems to provide universal access for the 70 million Americans—almost 30 percent of the population—who represent the society's future. An expansion of federal and state matching funds, as in Medicaid, along with employer coverage for collaborative school-based and health-plan services could yield at least a relative right for the initial decades. After years of attempting to address aspects of the problem, it appears that Americans might be ready to implement universal access to comprehensive health services for infants, children, and adolescents.

THE WORKING YEARS

The employer is the predominant source of third-party coverage. The similarity with government financing is suggested by the term *corporate socialism*, which some analysts use to describe this system of providing health benefits. A look at almost anyone's paycheck stub shows that the large gap between gross and net pay is accounted for by not only government but also "voluntary" taxation. The president's plan would make the provision of health benefits by all employers mandatory to ensure basic insurance coverage for full-time workers.

Coverage would include many of the health benefits now provided by large corporations. the traditional services of physicians and hospitals, outpatient care, laboratory studies, and prescription drugs. Preventive care, periodic medical exams, immunization, and screenings such as mammograms are being proposed. The costs of more generous benefits on the part of employers would be provided by taxable income.

Average premiums for the standard package are estimated at $1,800 per year for an individual and $4,200 for families. Employers would be responsible for 80 percent of the cost but could opt to pay more. Deductibles and copayment are proposed for high-cost plans, with out-of-pocket expenses capped at $1,500 per person and $3,000 per family. Business contributions would be capped at 7.9 percent of payroll. Small businesses with fewer than fifty employees would be eligible for government subsidies.

No health plan could deny enrollment to any person because of health status or lack of financial resources. In theory, the plans would reduce administrative costs and impose discipline largely through premium caps yielding a budget. Insurance would be obtained through regional health alliances established to collect premiums and negotiate coverage with health plans. States would ensure coverage for all communities. Companies with more than 5,000 employees could function as their own corporate alliances. Medicare would be phased into health alliances over time, and states would have the option of integrating Medicaid eligibles.

The issue of mandated benefits divides the corporate and small-business sectors of the country. Employees of large corporations receive health insurance as a tax-free benefit. Small operations view health benefits as an unreasonable or unfundable cost of doing business, and they provide limited, if any, coverage or subsidy. Since most jobs in the United States are in small businesses, the concerns of this group must be addressed. Although the goal is universal access to health care, the dramatic disparities between large corporations and the neighborhood cleaners, bakery, and shoe-repair shop would seem to argue for more customized strategies. Either coverage of cross-subsidization by insurance premiums or tax subsidies will be required.

Workers' compensation programs represent a major source of financing health care in the working years. State regulated, they are covered largely by third-party insurers using federal standards. The states' role and experience in this health-care program must be evaluated and exploited.

The Clinton administration's advocacy of mandated employer coverage, along with several proposals pending in the Congress, reflects a priority for the working years and the tradition of viewing health care as a fringe benefit of employment. The evolution of health-care financing through third parties spans six decades. Mandated coverage by employers for the working years of employees and their dependents represents an incremental next move. Health services for the initial decades and the retirement years, however, need financing that will foster and sustain creative if not heterodoxical restructuring of health care.

THE RETIREMENT YEARS

Despite the allocation of $129 billion for 35 million Americans ($3,686 per beneficiary) in 1992, Medicare is still not comprehensive.[6] It has not covered long-term care, out-of-pocket costs for prescription drugs, and copayments. But the elderly are better covered than the remainder of society, and it is more and more difficult to argue for the provision of additional special benefits. The societal right of health care for the elderly will be maintained. A means test can be applied, not at the point of provision of health care but through taxation of Social Security benefits and income-adjusted premiums for Medicare Part B. The financing will no doubt continue to include federal revenues, trust-fund contributions, out-of-pocket insurance premiums for Part B, and Medigap policies.

The disproportionate allocation of resources for the elderly is certain to become a significant political issue. The need of the elderly for health services is clearly greater than the need of other age cohorts. But the potential benefits or payoffs to society will be more if health services are augmented for children, youth, and the workforce.

Long-term care is unquestionably a major societal concern. Perhaps in no other area is the issue of health care as an absolute or relative right more problematic. The development of life-care communities has demonstrated the value of the community model of health services in supplementing and, on occasion, offsetting more traditional services. Long-term care of the elderly requires the conceptual model of nursing, with its functional and caring priorities, and that model, too, will become increasingly important in shaping strategies for this population group. There will be pressure to find trade-offs and lower-cost alternatives.

Long-term care is clearly an infinite need. The Medicare experience with the hospice concept is instructive, but the benefit for standard care of terminal illness is of arbitrary duration. The commitment for gerontology and long-term care is potentially too open-ended. It seems imperative to have decisions on resource allocation made by state and local communities using federal and state grants or fees paid to communities and institutions to develop programs and budgets.

Coverage of prescription drugs calls for especially innovative strategies. The cost of prescription drugs can drain a significant portion of a Social Security recipient's cash. More widespread reliance on bulk purchasing of drugs and a mail-order system of distribution are promising initiatives. Sustained creativity will be needed to develop cost-effective ways of providing this benefit.

One can approach health care for the elderly by influencing their perception of the need for services and their willingness to cope with the consequences of the aging process. Or one can attempt to ration the medical technology available in order to respond to their expressed needs. Any national roster of benefits and associated fee schedules is destined to focus on rationing.

Medicaid and Universal Access

A single-payer strategy or comprehensive mandated employer coverage for 260 million Americans would probably fix the health-care system in its present configuration for decades. This has been the experience of most other societies when they have implemented national health insurance. Health services for the young and the elderly in American society clearly require creative, flexible strategies if the country is to address infinite needs with finite resources. Medicaid, long a pariah of medical care, has the potential for becoming a proactive component of health-care reform for the initial and the retirement years.

A majority of the population is covered by third-party health insurance provided or subsidized by employers. Although not beneficiaries of Medicare, they are contributing toward the costs of benefits for the elderly and are aware of the program. Moreover, third-party insurance cross-subsidizes when Medicare pays less than costs. The third major player in health-care financing, Medicaid, is known to most Americans through reports, usually unfavorable, in newspapers and on television. Medicaid expenditures were estimated at $120 billion for 1992, having increased an average of 20 percent per year since 1989. Approximately two-thirds of the total was provided by the federal government.

When Medicaid was enacted in 1965, it authorized a benefit structure to include (1) inpatient hospital services, (2) outpatient hospital services, (3) laboratory and X-ray services, (4) skilled nursing-home services, (5) physician services, (6) other remedial care by licensed practitioners, (7) home health care, (8) private-duty nursing services, (9) clinical services, (10) dental services, (11) physical therapy and related services, (12) prescription drugs, dentures, eyeglasses, and prostheses, (13) other diagnostic screening, preventive, and rehabilitative services, (14) services at tuberculosis hospitals, mental hospitals, and skilled nursing homes for those sixty-five and older, and (15) other medical and remedial care recognized by state law. Although restricted to the elderly, children eighteen and under, mothers with dependent children, and medically indigent disabled persons, Medicaid offered a compelling precedent for comprehensive health services. The states, however, were passive players in the 1960s. Now they are proactive and aggressive.

Most states implemented Medicaid by placing the administrative responsibility in the welfare department. It was, after all, a means-tested benefit that required determination of eligibility, usually income measured as a percentage of the federal poverty level. Fluctuations in an individual's or family's income meant fluctuations in eligibility, a situation hardly conducive to continuity of health care. A number of states have subsequently recognized Medicaid as primarily a health-care program.

Medicaid is a major source for the payment of health services for infants, children, and pregnant women. It is estimated that almost a third of the nation's more than 4 million births in 1992 were covered by Medicaid. Moreover, 19 million children and youth under the age of twenty-one—a third of that segment of the population—were Medicaid beneficiaries at some time during the year, constituting half of all Medicaid beneficiaries.

At the other end of the age continuum, Medicaid is also a major source of funds for long-term care of the elderly. More than half the $60 billion expended on nursing-home care in 1991 came from public sources, chiefly Medicaid. When the need for long-term care is assessed, all of us are potentially medically indigent.

The initial and the retirement years require significant innovation in the organization, financing, and delivery of health services to address infinite needs with finite resources. When one contemplates the scale and depth of the problems, use of the states suggests a plausible initiative in reform. Can Medicaid be made more relevant, effective, and user-friendly? Certainly Medicaid focused on population segments could take us in the direction of entitlement to basic health services.

The Medicaid waiver to Oregon, for example, could go far beyond supporting that state's effort to allocate resources equitably among the poor. It could be a precedent for a comprehensive transformation of what is basically a welfare program into a health-care program. The principle of variable matching of state expenditures depending on the relative economic strength of the state is a principle found in a variety of programs. Subsidy by the federal government of initiatives at the state level has much merit. There is not only a decentralization of administrative responsibility but also a recognition of different problems and priorities. The approach could represent health-care restructuring through the states rather than only through a single payer or through employer mandate. Medicaid financing permits the use of waivers to pursue innovations appropriate to the care of children and youth and those people of retirement age.

Never until now has an overarching enactment in the United States attempted to address the total population as the British National Health Act did in 1946 and the Canadian Health Act in 1984. Most

American initiatives have focused on incremental priorities for segments of society. Much as the Founding Fathers, wary of a strong parliament, divided governmental powers among three branches, the country has kept health policy to a manageable scope and scale; its steps have been cautious to date.

The Quest for Health

The first principle of health-care reform—universal access—is easy to define: everyone would be covered. The second principle—development of a roster of core benefits—is more subjective, reflecting professional and personal priorities. Who defines the benefits for whom? And how does society finance core benefits for everyone? A universal entitlement paid for by a progressive federal income tax would in principle afford the most equity in health care. Such an entitlement would be patterned after Medicare or the Canadian health-insurance system. Even if that financing policy were achieved, the country would still be faced with establishing the mechanisms for resource allocation among varying health needs and alternative delivery systems. With a population of 260 million people drawn from more than a hundred ethnic backgrounds and distributed among fifty states covering 3.6 million square miles, the United States faces seemingly overwhelming societal challenges for access, quality, and cost containment.

During World War II the United States made the transition from a Depression to a robust economy. Independently and then collectively, several leaders sought to find ways to continue the economic vitality.[7] The Employment Act of 1946 created the Office of Economic Advisers in the White House and the Joint Economic Committee in Congress, but perhaps of greater significance, it established three goals for the American economy: "to promote maximum employment, production, and purchasing power."[8] All would agree that realization of these goals would promote the general welfare, but how? The executive, the legislator, and the economist, representing corporations, labor, and academe, argue over the merits of tax policy, fiscal policy, and monetary policy as the preferred mechanisms. Economic policy is an imprecise science. So, most certainly, is health policy.

To promote the general welfare and the health status of individuals while limiting expenditures to appropriate levels of resource consumption, I propose the following three goals, patterned after those of the Employment Act of 1946: guarantee access to appropriate health care for all Americans, maintain health-care expenditures at levels comparable to those of other economically advanced societies, and adjust expenditures to demographic changes and gains in cost and quality effectiveness. Even if there is agreement as to the ends, one can anticipate disagreement and vigorous debate as to the means.

The first goal resembles the societal commitment to a basic education. In education the commitment is measured in terms of years of input more than it is in levels of competence at completion. Realistically, at least in the foreseeable future, basic health services would be measured similarly—in terms of access rather than of health outcomes.

When no cost is too great to save a life or treat disease, efforts to achieve health care can be pursued at all costs if third-party coverage provided by the employer or the government eliminates market constraints. The goal to limit overall expenditures to the level achieved in other competitively advanced societies is the equivalent of the goal to "promote purchasing power," that is, to control inflation.

Finally, population growth and greater intensity of care each account for a third of the annual increases in health expenditures. Investments in cost-effectiveness to address increases in health-care expenditures are imperative.

Whatever measures of reform are advocated, legislated, or implemented, the health-care enterprise will be challenged for decades to come by the health-system equivalents of tax, fiscal, and monetary policy. The principles of a preferred strategy are discussed in the next chapter.

Chapter 11
Hang Together or
Hang Separately

To manage, or to be managed,
that is the question.

The Constitution advances the values central to the American experience. The separation of the powers of government expresses the American suspicion of monolithic strategies; the First Amendment guarantees of freedom of religion, speech, and assembly convey the country's pluralism. But as Ben Franklin told his colleagues at the signing of the Declaration of Independence, "We must all hang together, or assuredly we shall all hang separately." The determination of the colonies to be bound through the Articles of Confederation and the Constitution provided an alternative to hanging separately. Can the American experience offer the same alternative in the health-care enterprise?

The tradition of voluntary community hospitals begun when Ben Franklin founded the Pennsylvania Hospital in 1751 has flourished for two and a half centuries and finds contemporary expression in several thousand local and regional institutions. Can physicians hang together by entering into joint ventures with the community hospitals in which they now serve as voluntary staff members? Preferred provider organizations (PPOS) and their multiple variations seem to anticipate the transition from fee for service and solo practice to the organized practice of medicine using equitable prepayment.[1] I believe the future is with health-care systems. The questions are what kind, how they should be organized, and what ends they will serve.

Health-care systems emphasize the inextricable relations between financing and organization in facilitating delivery of services. The American health-care enterprise includes an abundance of initiatives and experiments in the organization and delivery of health services that is unequaled in the world. From relatively small, decentralized medical society–sponsored independent practice associations (IPAS) to the Kaiser Foundation Health Plan, the spectrum includes horizontal multi-institutional hospital systems and vertically integrated systems linking primary, secondary, and tertiary levels of care.[2] The pluralism and pragmatism, of the American character suggest that strategies for health will be forged by associations that evolve from solo practice and voluntary-staffed community hospitals to the organized practice of medicine sustained by prepayment.

The Ben Franklin Scenario

Health-care systems range from very loose affiliations to unitary organizations, each offering a variety of constraints and incentives for the participants. In what I call the Ben Franklin scenario because it reflects a determination to "hang together," six principles are operative: consumer-provider choice, enrolled population, community-weighted capitation, organized practice, prospective budgets, and cost-effective health-care (fig. 9). These principles, discussed below, represent aspirations, not requirements. In certain areas of the country, population characteristics, resource constraints, and established traditions of health care would require modification of one or the other principle. The Ben Franklin scenario is almost fully operative in some health-care systems, while it functions only partially in others.

CONSUMER-PROVIDER CHOICE

The opportunity to choose is fundamental in American society. Ray E. Brown, a leading hospital administrator, points out that

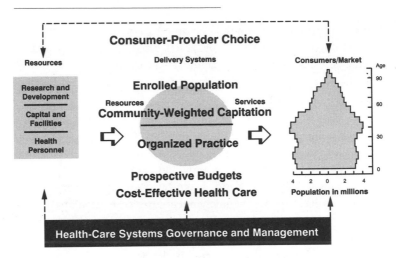

Fig. 9. The Ben Franklin Scenario

"in the United States, we select hospitals not by virtue of residence, as we do schools, but rather by choice, as we do churches."[3] He implies both the voluntary character of medical institutions and their close link with American values. The evaluation of health care is highly subjective, an extension of one's culture and beliefs. Moreover, the outcomes of health care are often not as desired by the consumer or the provider. Movement from one type of provider to another can be a safety valve for frustration on the part of the patient. Increasingly, consumer choice is an element in employee health-benefit coverage. The patient needs a range of manageable choices but something less than the free choice represented by all the listings of physicians in the Yellow Pages of the local telephone directory.

For the provider, choice can enhance professional satisfaction. The personal nature of health services makes it desirable that the providers have choice and be committed to the systems in which they function. Individual practitioners' priorities vary. For some physicians medicine is a calling, for others primarily an intellectual challenge, and for others a service transaction. All of them can be productive and effective in the appropriate environments.

ENROLLED POPULATION

Health care has a population, as well as an individual, dimension. A number of strategies, such as immunization, benefit from both a population and an individual focus. As concerns for health promotion and disease prevention increase, strategies in a group context will be more important. The health needs of a changing and aging population confronting finite resources will require increasing attention to community strategies that synthesize medical care, public health, and social welfare much as they do for the young. An enrolled population also provides a basis for stable funding and allocation planning commensurate with anticipatory strategies. Every citizen must have the opportunity to enroll in a health-care system of his or her choice.

COMMUNITY-WEIGHTED CAPITATION

Prepayment of health services began in 1929 with the concept of community rating: each schoolteacher in Dallas, Texas, paid fifty cents a month as a deposit to ensure the availability of hospital services if needed. Community rating was eroded by experience rating as commercial insurance companies sought to carve out a market niche in a lucrative and expanding postwar health-care economy. If the cost of health care is to be covered in an equitable fashion, a return to some variation of community rating is imperative. In community-weighted capitation, each individual would pay, or have paid for him or her, a monthly premium adjusted for, or weighted by, a few selected variables based on age and an index of broad morbidity experience. Medicare risk contracts currently represent community-weighted capitation. The total payment up front to the health-care delivery system would be determined by the number of enrollees accepted. Community-weighted capitation continues the society's tradition of cross-subsidization.

ORGANIZED PRACTICE

The solo practice of medicine has benefits for those with enough time and money. But any attempt to achieve health care, even as a relative right, for 260 million Americans will require that random medicine be a limited experience—probably representing less than a quarter of all health services. While advocating organized practice for the vast majority, I would defend the opportunity to pay for unlimited choice as an option and a safety valve.

The form of organized practice can vary. Partnerships, single-specialty groups, and multispecialty groups abound, as do groups of outpatient and emergency-room staffs, hospital-based radiology and anesthesiology groups, neighborhood health centers, and large group practices. Some existing preferred provider organizations and hospital-physician joint ventures will probably evolve into new forms. Overall, the experimentation and pragmatism that have characterized many of the developments in the American health-care enterprise ought to provide new and unique systems.

PROSPECTIVE BUDGETS

Diagnostic-related groups were adopted by the federal government as a vehicle for shifting Medicare financing of hospitals from retrospective cost-based reimbursement to prospective case-based payment. Aggregation of services as specific DRGs and the substitution of prospective payment for retrospective reimbursement meant developing a budget for the hospital. The usual strategy for addressing infinite needs with finite resources is to set priorities in a prospective budget. Health-care systems must acknowledge that limited resources have to be budgeted. The array of services sought must be delivered, substituted for, or deferred. The choice would appear to be between prospective rationalization through allocation of resources or retrospective rationing. Budgeting by a health-care system represents the preferred choice.

COST-EFFECTIVE HEALTH CARE

Cost-effectiveness, or cost benefit, is the most compelling argument for the pluralism of the Ben Franklin scenario. Analyses of cost-effectiveness, while utilizing scientific and statistical methods, incorporate subjective assumptions. Selection of the benefits—a choice of values—determines the calculation. Quality is now being recognized by providers as their first goal, and numerous health-care systems in the United States are pursuing the principles of total quality management (TQM) or continuous quality improvement (CQI).[4] Total quality management recognizes the ultimate aspiration of cost-effectiveness by addressing every dimension of the provision of a service and the relative contributions to quality outcomes.

Prototypes for Health-Care Reform

The most significant achievements in cost-effective health care will be realized when all the principles of the Ben Franklin scenario are in play. In my experience, three health-care systems best approximate the scenario. Each offers an example for health-care reforms.

HENRY FORD HEALTH SYSTEM

Using both the Mayo Clinic and the Johns Hopkins Hospital as models, Henry Ford took over the Detroit General Hospital Project in 1915. The Henry Ford Health System has expanded beyond a 900-bed teaching hospital to include four hospitals with a total of 1,600 beds, thirty-five outpatient centers, and six twenty-four-hour emergency facilities in four counties surrounding Detroit. Currently, the Henry Ford Medical Group comprises 900 physicians. Henry Ford Health System developed the nation's ninth-largest HMO, Health Alliance Plan, which has 450,000 members (40 percent of southeastern Michigan's HMO market), utilizing its own 120-member medical group and 1,500 affiliated community physicians. The system is Michigan's eighth-largest employer, retaining a professional and support staff of 15,500.

Total revenues in 1992 were $1.270 billion. The largest portion of the system's revenues is HMO capitation. The second-largest portion is Medicare, followed by Blue Cross/Blue Shield and commercial insurance. The Henry Ford Foundation endowment provides a significant amount of capital for expansion efforts and program development. The market value of the fund was $184 million at the end of 1992.[5]

Henry Ford Health System is dedicated to developing and providing the highest-quality health care to serve the needs of the southeastern Michigan community. Supported by nationally recognized education and research programs, the system's services seek to be the most comprehensive, efficient, and clinically effective in the region.

GROUP HEALTH COOPERATIVE OF PUGET SOUND

A coalition of consumers, business executives, and union members in the Seattle area, concerned about the economic threat of illness at the end of World War II, incorporated in 1947 as the Group Health Cooperative of Puget Sound, selling memberships in a non-profit health-care plan for $100. The clinical service began with a fifteen-physician Medical Security Clinic, which owned a fifty-five bed hospital.[6]

Today, almost a half-century later, Group Health Cooperative of Puget Sound is a recognized leader among staff-model HMOs. Its enrollment approaches 500,000, making it the seventh-largest nonprofit HMO in the country. The original group of sixteen physicians has grown to more than 750 full-time-equivalent physicians and other medical staff and almost 900 full-time-equivalent staff nurses, who provide health services at thirty primary-care or family medical centers, five specialty medical centers, two hospitals, an inpatient-care center, and a skilled-nursing facility. Community partners are utilized in other areas. Revenues for 1992 were $854 million.

Group Health has developed strategies in pursuit of the best possible clinical outcomes for its enrollees. These clinical road maps, as they are called, are interdisciplinary endeavors to identify, describe, and define appropriate care; test and improve current systems; and evaluate services. Teams are underway to provide prenatal care, diabetes management, assistance in stopping smoking, and other selected health-care services. Each initiative exploits the several principles of the Ben Franklin scenario in the synthesis of medical care and the proactive strategies of public health.

KAISER PERMANENTE MEDICAL PROGRAM

In 1992, the Kaiser Foundation Health Plan cared for 6.6 million enrollees with 9,000 physicians and annual revenues of $11 billion. Headquartered in Oakland, California, this prototype of a group-model HMO originated on the West Coast over fifty years ago and now has a nationwide presence in sixteen states, from Hawaii to Colorado, Ohio, Connecticut, Washington, D.C., North Carolina, Georgia, and Texas. Kaiser Permanente is the largest nongovernmental health-care delivery system in the world. Kaiser (the business side) and Permanente (the medical side) work as partners to provide prepaid medical care. The fourteen Kaiser Permanente Medical Groups range in size from 45,000 to 2.5 million subscribers.[7]

The Kaiser Permanente Medical Program pursues the implementation of seven basic principles: preventive care and health promotion, joint physician responsibility for program management and effectiveness, prepayment, multispecialty group practice, organized facilities and service, voluntary enrollment and consumer choice, and nonprofit status. The principles, developed in the 1930s by Kaiser's pioneer, Dr. Sidney Garfield, represent a "genetic code" for many of his successors.

Hypothetically, thirty-eight Kaisers could provide all the primary and secondary, and some of the tertiary, medical care required for a population of 260 million Americans at approximately 46 percent of the current total cost and with less than half the physicians practicing medicine in the United States. This would be the equivalent of expanding the National Football League from 28 to 1,064 teams. Admittedly, the Kaiser population is not a representative sample of the United States population; nor is Kaiser prominent in long-term care or related service. Without attempting a detailed analysis of demographics and socioeconomic characteristics, I would suggest that the equivalent of at least sixty Kaisers, modified for specific requirements and circumstances, would be required to do the job. The scale of the challenge would be formidable, even for health-care reform.

These three prototypes combine organization of health personnel with capitation financing in pursuit of cost-effectiveness. The independent practice association, pioneered by the San Joaquin Medical Care Foundation in the 1950s as a competitor to Kaiser in California, seeks to preserve the autonomy of medical practice in the Ben Franklin scenario. Two rapidly growing IPAs close to home in Philadelphia illustrate some 60 percent of the HMO experience.

U.S. Healthcare, headquartered near Philadelphia, is one of the largest for-profit HMOs in the country, with over 1.6 million subscribers in Pennsylvania, New Jersey, Delaware, and New York. The company had revenues of $1.3 billion in 1990 and 2.2 billion in 1992. Approximately 6,000 primary-care physicians each enroll a minimum goal of 500 patients, for whom they receive monthly capitation payments. A roster of 19,000 specialists, reimbursed on a fee-for-service basis from budgeted pools of funds, is available on referral. Specialist fees and hospital contracts are negotiated by the plan, which is at risk for their utilization. U.S. Healthcare has pioneered physician incentives for quality healthcare and outcome measure.[8]

Keystone Health is an IPA operated by Independence Blue Cross and Pennsylvania Blue Shield. This HMO has a membership of 550,000, approximately one-third of whom are Medicaid beneficiaries. The plan contracts with 5,500 physicians and sixty hospitals for the provision of health services. Blue Cross and Blue Shield, the pioneers in third-party health insurance in the 1930s, now pursue alternative strategies for the organization, financing, and delivery of health services. In Philadelphia these include a variety of approaches to health-care reform, including Personal Choice—a point-of-service plan—and the development of a staff-model HMO.[9]

Other prototypes of the Ben Franklin scenario can be identified across the country: Health Insurance Plan of Greater New York, Geisinger Clinic, Harvard Community Health Care Plan, Group Health of Washington, D.C., Community Health Center Plan in New Haven, and Genesee Community Health Plan, to list a few. These are among some 550 health maintenance organizations that serve populations ranging from tens of thousands to more than a million.

During a career spanning three decades I have visited more than 500 health-care institutions and systems in forty-six states. None is perfect, many are exemplary, and no two are identical. Many are pursuing two or more of the principles of the Ben Franklin scenario. When one surveys health care in the United States, it is evident that, if there are five ways of doing something, all five ways are being used and someone is looking for a sixth.

To Manage or to Be Managed

The Ben Franklin scenario is elegant in its simplicity but awesome in its complexity. The expectations of both the provider and the consumer are but two dimensions of the complexities. The financial and accounting gymnastics required to survive in health care make it a wonder that the American system devotes only a quarter of its expenditures to administration. It is to be hoped that nurses and physicians would recognize this complexity and see weighted capitation as an opportunity to shift costs from administration to clinical services.

The organized practice of medicine, once regarded as anathema, now seems possible. In the broadest terms, capitated payment represents a synthesis of medical practice and public health, incorporating anticipatory strategies, population-based accountability, budgeting, and organized practice. Each of the resultant delivery systems must address the tension between excellence and equity while controlling costs.

The strength of the Marcus Welby scenario was in physician autonomy, prerogative, and authority. In an effort to preserve fee for service and solo practice, however, physicians are paying the price of bureaucratic constraints and red tape. To quote Gilbert and Sullivan's *Pirates of Penzance*, "A paradox? A paradox, a most ingenious paradox." The very ingredients of the Lilliputian scenario that threaten the autonomy, prerogative, and authority of the physician can become the instruments of self-control and total quality management as the "managee" becomes the manager in the Ben Franklin scenario. One person's red tape becomes coordination for others. The physician's autonomy, prerogative, and authority are replaced by the health-care system's autonomy, prerogative, and authority.

Prior authorization can be pursued proactively by a health-care system instead of functioning as a last-minute barrier or mandated clearance. Health-care systems have developed varying strategies and policies for resource allocation and distribution of services within delivery systems. These represent de facto anticipatory prior authorization, in which those responsible for providing the services participate in the decision making and the determination of priorities.

Second opinion, imposed by edict in some managed-care strategies, has long been realized in the "corridor consultations" so highly valued in community hospitals and group practices. The more the decision to seek a second opinion is part of the physician-patient interaction and the more responsive it is to policies and strategies designed by the providers responsible for delivering the services, the more likely it is to enhance outcomes.

Utilization review and related mechanisms for quality assessment are increasingly prominent in health-care systems. Some systems use methodologies and databases developed by research institutes or consulting firms. Others, such as the Harvard Community Health Plan, have built a management culture around evaluation of utilization and quality. Total quality management and continuous quality improvement play roles in a number of systems, notably Henry Ford Health System, Group Health Cooperative, and Kaiser Permanente.

Diagnostic-related groups were developed to address the internal interface of medicine, nursing, and management. And that is the area where DRGs belong. They have great potential for systems evaluation and utilization review, but as instruments of macro–health policy for the purpose of resource allocation, they simply tighten the bonds on the Gulliver-like physician.

Resource-based/relative-value scales probably have the greatest potential for constraining physicians committed to fee for service and solo practice. With expenditures for physicians' services under Medicare Part B running out of control, the Health Care Financing Administration and the Department of Health and Human Services had to do something. Physician DRGs were considered. There is no mechanism for compensating physicians that is simultaneously responsive to the best interests of the patient; the institution, community, or society; and the physician. Health-care systems can design suitable payment mechanisms, evaluate them, and make changes without waiting for an act of Congress.

Therapeutic protocols will be the likely form of practice guidelines. The question will be who designs them and for whom. Protocols are absolutely essential for certain biomedical technologies. The Ben Franklin scenario allows for broader, more intimate participation of physicians than a central determination by the Health Care Financing Administration would. Therapeutic protocols developed by a group of peers in the context of total quality management and closely monitored for clinical outcomes could become an asset rather than just so much red tape.

Thus the instruments of cost containment in managed care become the mechanisms for pursuing cost-effectiveness in the Ben Franklin scenario. Hospital-physician joint ventures, preferred provider organizations, and managed-care initiatives will evolve along the lines of the Ben Franklin scenario or they will be controlled centrally by the Lilliputian scenario (see table 9). As Hamlet might have said, to manage, or to be managed, that is the question.

From Primary Care to Tertiary Care

The Ben Franklin scenario focuses on primary and secondary care. Primary care is widely discussed, but what is secondary care? Some conclude somewhat cynically that secondary care is primary care provided by a tertiary specialist. Actually, though, primary care and tertiary care anchor the opposite poles of comprehensive health services, with secondary care constituting the middle ground.

Primary care comprises most health care. The next stage of the continuum is classified as either primary or secondary, depending on whether the services are provided by a generalist—a family physician, general internist, or nurse practitioner—or a specialist such as a gastroenterologist, allergist, or endocrinologist. The overlap of professional competence is confusing and often leads to such debates as whether a colonoscopy is better performed by a gastroenterologist, an internist, or a general surgeon. Diagnostic and therapeutic technological tools like X-ray machines, automated blood analyzers, sonography, lasers, not to mention tens of thousands of highly potent and sophisticated drugs, however, are available to virtually all practitioners.

Table 9
To Manage or to Be Managed

Ben Franklin Scenario	Lilliputian Scenario
Consumer-provider choice	Prior authorization
Enrolled population	Second opinion
Community-weighted capitation	Utilization review
Organized practice	Diagnostic-related groups
Prospective budgets	Resource-based/relative-value scales
Cost-effective health care	Therapeutic protocols

Tertiary care occurs farther along on the continuum, where definitions become more precise and agreement on categories of care more complete. Heart transplants, liver transplants, chemotherapy and radiation for cancer, bone-marrow transplants, PET scanning, and selective intensive care with physiological monitoring qualify as tertiary care. These services are provided predominantly in university medical centers and referral centers but are also spun off to larger community hospitals. The entrepreneurial spirit that encourages each hospital to acquire the latest in sophisticated technology has been called a biomedical arms race.

Many of America's economic competitors guarantee access to primary care but ration tertiary care. Since American society prefers to deny that it rations, what will be an acceptable mechanism for resource allocation? In the Ben Franklin scenario, health-care systems in urban and surrounding areas will be able to provide primary and secondary health care to populations of 300,00 to 500,000. Larger health-care systems, such as Kaiser, and those with referral bases similar to Henry Ford's will provide an amalgam of primary, secondary, and some tertiary care. In rural areas, on the other hand, those seeking to implement the Ben Franklin scenario with enrollments of 10,000 to 50,000 will require backup simply to provide secondary care. The vast majority of health-care systems in the Ben Franklin scenario will need to establish linkages to provide tertiary care.

There are two basic alternatives for organizing a continuum of health services: referral to selected specialists or institutions on contract for services or participation in a defined regional network. Either alternative can operate effectively. As national health policy, both should continue to be developed. Variations on these themes are certain to be implemented.

How should two- or three-tiered comprehensive health-care systems be organized? Who should select or designate tertiary-care centers? Some analysts advocate the forces of the market. Others prefer public-sector control. The Mayo Clinic, the Cleveland Clinic, and Johns Hopkins Medical Center are private not-for-profit referral centers with a national and international clientele. The University of Iowa Hospital and Clinics is the tax-supported tertiary-care base for an entire state.

The contractual approach is adaptable to existing institutional and practice patterns. Moreover, it is flexible and incremental. Although duplication and inefficiency are possible, the services can be highly individualized. For example, an internist at York Hospital in Pennsylvania can refer a cardiac patient to Johns Hopkins in Baltimore, a cancer patient to the University of Pennsylvania in Philadelphia, and a neurologic patient to the Cleveland Clinic. This approach provides the freedom of choice so highly esteemed in American society. Moreover, competition and negotiated contracts often help contain costs.

The regional medical programs legislated in 1965 authorized planning and operational grants to develop cooperative arrangements among medical schools, hospitals, and physicians. Fifty-six regions within and across state lines were organized to establish patient referral networks and continuing-education linkages. The University of Missouri replicated the model of the extension service to provide physicians with technological support for diagnostic studies. The Connecticut regional medical program enabled the medical centers of Yale and the University of Connecticut to affiliate with community hospitals throughout the state for subspecialty referral, residency training, and student rotations. The University of Iowa Hospital and Clinics emphasized linkages for postgraduate medical education and collaborative clinical research. Only a few regional medical programs, however, attempted significant changes in the care system.

Everett Dirksen of Illinois, the Senate minority leader during the New Frontier and the Great Society, was fond of citing the adage that no army can withstand the strength of an idea whose time has come. Many of us thought that regional medical programs were just such an idea when President Johnson signed the legislation enacting them. History proved us wrong. We underestimated the complexity of the concept and the difficulty of articulating it. The legislation was allowed to expire in 1974 after nine years of limited achievement and mixed reviews. Participants at a twenty-fifth-anniversary symposium discussed whether the problem was the idea or the timing, especially as developments of the past three decades suggest the society is moving inexorably toward regional medical programs once again. [10]

The development of health systems, the initiatives of health maintenance organizations, and the emergence of health-services research on a major scale provide the ingredients for creating regional medical programs that link university medical centers, biomedical and health-services research institutions (experimental stations), systems demonstrations (model farms), and outreach and continuing education (extension services). This time the idea would not be subverted by the costly efforts of Medicare and Medicaid to preserve the Marcus Welby scenario.

Much as Johns Hopkins served in 1889 as the prototype for the Flexnerian model that has shaped medical education in the United States for a century, its current health system can be seen as one of the prototypes for a vertically integrated system based on an academic health center. The University of Pennsylvania Health System is being developed as an accountable health plan spanning primary to tertiary care. Allegheny Health Systems in Pittsburgh has acquired two medical schools in Philadelphia. A diversity of other initiatives can be anticipated as health-care reform is implemented in the private, independent, and public sectors.

In the Ben Franklin scenario, some institutions will be large enough to incorporate the resources to provide tertiary care. Most will either refer patients to selected institutions or participate in networks of strategic alliances. At the rate that hospitals, groups of physicians, and the other parties in health care are scrambling to hang together, it would appear that they subscribe to the wisdom of another of Franklin's aphorisms—"You may delay, but time will not."

Chapter 12
Health Care for the
Twenty-first Century

Medicine discovers the future.
Management seeks a preferred future.

When President Clinton presented his proposal for health-care reform to a joint session of Congress on 22 September 1993, few disagreed that the American health system is badly in need of fixing. His prescription was expressed in terms of six principles: Security (universal coverage of comprehensive health benefits), simplicity (reduction in insurance red tape), savings (reduction in premium increases and administrative costs), quality (standards for services and outcome measures), choice (fee-for-service, point-of-service, or managed care), and responsibility (consumer participation in purchases and alternative approaches to malpractice, fraud, and abuse). The details, laid out in a 284-page book entitled *The President's Health Security Plan*, constitute a strategy for a pervasive restructuring of the American health-care system, an enterprise equivalent to the world's eighth-largest economy.[1] The proposed legislative reform submitted to the Congress five weeks later as the 1,342-page *Health Security Act* describes a social experiment on an unprecedented scale.

Can the proposed managed competition master the iron triangle of

149

health care—access, quality, and cost containment—through health alliances and accountable health plans? Can the behemoth of the American health-care enterprise be subject to the all-encompassing embrace of a national health board and a global budget? Will the American people accept such trade-offs as relative access, increased waiting times, or limitations on the latest technology?

As a medical student I learned an important lesson: when a patient has a host of pathologies or multi-organ-systems disease, selective therapeutic strategies are critical. Any attempt to treat everything at once risks a confluence of physiological and pharmacological side effects that could overwhelm the patient; one has to address specifics and to anticipate consequences. My experience suggests that the same holds true for health-care systems. Comprehensive reform, while attractive in theory, is a high-risk venture.

The more extensive the restructuring of health care sought and the more accelerated the legislative process, the more formidable the challenges that must be addressed by implementation in the decades ahead. The scope of any health-policy action determines the scale of the reciprocal overreaction, witness the consequences of the failure in Medicare to anticipate the inflationary trends in technology, demography, and utilization. Health-care reform appears to ignore three critical realities. While needs are infinite, resources are finite; the iron triangle of health care cannot be ignored. Societal entitlements are relative, not absolute. Finally, health-care values derive from our society's cultural pluralism, which cannot be ignored in determining benefit structure. Efforts must be made to avoid damaging the exemplary in health care.

Priorities for addressing these realities are better formulated by local health plans and the communities they serve than by monolithic strategies promulgated by a national health board. Aspirations and targets must, of course, relate to broad national health goals. However, control over the selection of the means for their realization must be placed close to where the services are provided. Markets may not work effectively in health care; nevertheless, consumer and provider choice in the transactions are imperative.

It must be emphasized that significant health-care reform is already under way. One can look at Hawaii as it approaches two decades of experience in implementing its version of national health insurance. Minnesota, the site of extensive private-sector initiatives, has enacted legislation for universal access. The state of Washington targets implementation of health-care reform through 1999. Rochester, New York, and Cleveland, Ohio, are pursuing significant, although different, approaches. *Fortune* 500 corporations, major health-insurance carriers, the Blues, and a variety of health-care systems are evolving into health alliances and accountable health plans.

Providing universal access to a standard benefit package of quality health care while controlling costs will require a well-balanced top-down, bottom-up collaboration. Cost containment or a global budget would be the concern of a national health board and regional alliances. Access to comprehensive health services must be the concern of community-grounded health plans at the base of the endeavor. Implementation will require incrementalism that appreciates precedent, pragmatism, and—above all—the society's cultural pluralism. Having worked in southern West Virginia, eastern Kentucky, rural New Mexico, and northern California, as well as in Philadelphia, Detroit, and the Bronx, I have a keen sense of America's diversity and the imperatives of pluralism.

Implementation of reform will undoubtedly test the Ben Franklin scenario. The Lilliputian scenario will most likely be played out by health alliances, while health plans commit themselves to the development of the Ben Franklin scenario. Health alliances, in efforts to contain costs, will seek vigorous implementation of managed care and the manipulation of health services that is inherent in trying to regulate and control providers. Health plans must seize the initiative for self-regulation and develop cost-effective services. After all, health-care systems are where the action is: there's where a patient encounters a physician or a nurse practitioner. The task of health-care reform must be to restrain the Lilliputians while facilitating the effort of the Ben Franklins.

Legislation and the Art of the Possible

When President Clinton held up a Health Security card before the joint session of Congress and the national television audience, he may have signaled phase one of health-care reform. Security, meaning guaranteed access, was his first principle. Any effort to guarantee access to health care for 260 million Americans in the near future, however, would compromise quality and cost containment. Access phased in incrementally, beginning with limited benefits, could be feasible.

My Social Security card is identical to my wife's. Mine carries significantly greater benefits because my full-time participation in the workforce has been three times hers. When we reach sixty-five, however, our Medicare benefits will be identical. The challenge to Congress in the short term is to launch the Health Security card along the lines of Social Security with a commitment to a phased implementation of the equity of Medicare.

Any legislation implementing health-care reform must address the question of who gives as well as the question of who receives. Security, choice, and quality all cost money and must be paid for. The President's *Health Security Plan* emphasizes the third-party strategy by mandating employer and employee contributions. A single-payer approach patterned after the Medicare trust fund is advocated by almost a hundred members of the House of Representatives. Tax deductions and tax credits for those most in need are also featured in legislative proposals. The individuals most in need of guaranteed access are the approximately 40 million Americans who are young or unemployed, who earn low wages, or who have been dropped from Medicaid. Their requirements could be approached with a phased benefit structure.

There are other reform initiatives that the Congress can address in the short term for incremental implementation into the long term. As noted, health care for infants, children, and pregnant women requires innovation in organization, financing, and delivery systems. Amendment, adaptation, and expansion of existing statutes could begin the transition to universal coverage for the future generation of American society.

Medicaid waivers have been used by Arizona and Oregon to move incrementally toward universal access to health care. This vehicle should be encouraged for other states. Some, such as Montana and Vermont, might apply this federal-state match and subsidy toward a single-payer strategy. Others could develop community-based programs for long-term care of the elderly.

Medicare and Medicaid are favorite targets for cost savings—$124 billion in the former and $65 billion in the latter over five years. The almost $75 billion per year in tax-exempt health benefits warrants equal consideration.

Virtually all the proposals before the 103rd Congress call for cost containment through reform of administrative duplication, fraud, abuse, and malpractice. The first, because it would mean simplification of forms, will make the most sense to the electorate.

Efforts to realize a global budget would require an orchestration of market, regulatory, and public-sector forces reminiscent of the ongoing interplay of monetary, fiscal, and tax policies addressed in the Employment Act of 1946. Accordingly, a council of health advisers patterned after the Council of Economic Advisers and a joint Senate-House health committee could be a preferable start toward a national health board.

Politics is the art of the possible. And what is possible for health-care reform in the 103rd Congress? Hearings to consider the vested interests of all the stakeholders in health care, let alone to encompass the jurisdictions of a significant number of the standing committees addressed in the *Health Security Act*, would bring new meaning to the notion of a herculean endeavor. Yet the process is prologue to findings, deliberation, report, debate, and enactment. On the other hand, members of the 103rd Congress, except for two-thirds of the senators, must face the electorate on 8 November 1994. Given the administration's commitment to, and the media's preoccupation with, health-care reform, senators and representatives can hardly approach the hustings empty-handed. Medicine's dilemmas become Congress's dilemmas, those of addressing infinite needs with finite resources.

Given the expectations of the public, as recorded in Louis Harris's January 1993 opinion poll, incremental measures that can be achieved in the short run must be seen as symbols of a commitment to significant health-care reform over the long haul. Those members who return to the 104th Congress will have a full agenda for two years. Even if universal access as a relative entitlement is enacted by the 103rd or

104th or a subsequent Congress, the 90 percent of the effort required for implementation will remain ahead of us.

The Momentum for Health-Care Reform

The President's Health Security Plan calls for the states to establish health alliances between 1995 and 1997, but implementation of reform will be a challenge for decades. A number of forces already present or operative will shape that reform: health care as an information industry, biomedical breakthroughs, patients as constituents, capitation and community-weighted rating, prospective budgets and resource allocation, management and the organized practice of medicine, adaptation of disciplines, professional education as a continuum, physicians' participation as citizens, and the synthesis of medicine and public health.

HEALTH CARE AS AN INFORMATION INDUSTRY

Health-care professionals collect, interpret, categorize, store, retrieve, analyze, and apply information. The classic information document is a patient's hospital chart, containing physicians' and nurses' notes, laboratory results, X-ray interpretations, and other relevant data. These observations and perspectives are now facilitated by computers; while the physician and the nurse may forget, the computer never does. Conversely, nurses and physicians are adept at creative thinking and intuition. Health care as an information industry demands new collaboration between technology and the human brain.

Physicians value their privileged communication with patients. They often feel their privacy, as well as that of the patient, has been violated when medical records are subpoenaed. Hospitals have felt the same protectiveness about data they collect on morbidity, mortality, complication rates, and so forth. Now the Health Care Financing Administration publishes these data.[2] The Freedom of Information Act may have a greater impact on health affairs than do a year's worth of articles in the *New England Journal of Medicine*.

Prescriptions were once written in Latin to convey information from physician to pharmacist. Now information on drugs is conveyed directly to the consumer in the print and television advertisements of pharmaceutical companies. Advertising influences not only over the counter sales but physicians' choices of specific companies' products.

The sovereign profession of medicine, as exemplified by Dr. Marcus Welby, owed much of its authority to control over its body of knowledge. Now that knowledge is being shared with the patient and the citizenry at large. The character of the patient-physician relationship is shifting.

BIOMEDICAL BREAKTHROUGHS

The marvels of modern biomedical science are perhaps nowhere more dramatically seen than in the discovery of polio vaccine. Dropping sugar cubes soaked with vaccine into the mouths of young children, as opposed to subjecting polio victims to creaking, heaving iron-lung machines, provided a powerful benefit—quality of life. Would that all scientific discoveries boasted as remarkable a cost-benefit ratio.

Chronic renal dialysis represents an intermediate technology for prolonging life—a life of diminished quality and significant suffering. Although the alternative is death, dialysis is a far cry from life-preserving polio vaccine. Moreover, the vaccine costs only a few cents to produce and a few dollars to distribute through organized public-health campaigns; chronic renal dialysis can cost $30,000 to $35,000 a year.[3]

As scientific efforts to map the human genome proceed at a robust pace, one must wonder about the implications. Will gene therapy replicate the polio miracle or the renal dialysis dilemma? The side effects of therapy, as well as the benefits, must bear on societal decisions on biomedical advances.

PATIENTS AS CONSTITUENTS

Late one evening during my internship at the Yale–New Haven Hospital, a surgical-ward nurse entered the office where I was catching up on patients' charts. An airline stewardess before attending nursing school, she asked, "Dr. Kissick, would you please look in on the passenger in the room at the end of the hall?" Her slip of the tongue was not entirely without basis. After all, airline passengers, like patients, are in the hands of professionals; physicians, like pilots, are clear about their destinations. Today the parallel can be carried further: passengers choose airlines rather than pilots, and patients have come to choose health-care systems rather than physicians.

Patients have become subscribers and beneficiaries. Increasingly one hears the term *consumer* as a counterpoint to *provider*. I like to call patients and potential patients *constituents*, a word connoting reciprocal accountability between the individuals seeking care and those providing services. Providers are accountable to their constituents, and their constituents, in turn, have an obligation to collaborate with them.

CAPITATION AND COMMUNITY-WEIGHTED RATING

Capitation, a predetermined monthly allocation to the health-care system on behalf of each individual or enrolled family, ensures the subscriber of coverage and the provider of earnings to cover services. Physicians and hospitals have the responsibility of generating budgets and determining priorities for resource allocation.

Medicare risk contracts calculate prepayment that is weighted to reflect age. The word *risk* is relative, as Medicare patients host a plethora of chronic diseases, and Medicare capitation rates exceed rates for younger, working populations. The challenge to any delivery system, however, is to provide cost-effective health services while avoiding high-tech alternatives with limited long-term utility.

PROSPECTIVE BUDGETS AND RESOURCE ALLOCATION

The term *prospective budgets* is redundant in a sense. It connotes, however, a budget developed from capitation payments and used as the basis for derivative strategies of resource allocation. The prospective budget is the transition force for addressing infinite needs with finite resources.

To avoid rationing, American society must adopt resource allocation. Where the British National Health Service admits to rationing, the American system pursues its rationing reactively and often in the glare of the media. The society creates a myth to cover ad hoc mechanisms that ignore equity for the almost 40 million people who are disenfranchised while they promise excellence to the rest. Budgeting seems antithetical to health care, yet the laws of economics are as relevant to health care as are the laws of molecular biology.

MANAGEMENT AND THE ORGANIZED PRACTICE OF MEDICINE

The corporate practice of medicine has been coming for about half a century. American medicine will not be dominated by corporations per se; rather it will experience a synthesis of the management sciences and the medical sciences. Cost-effective medicine will not, and probably cannot, be practiced free of management.

A creative synthesis of the professional model and a management model is imperative in health services characterized by pluralism, pragmatism, and principle. A dynamic approach requires research, development, testing, and evaluation in a goal-oriented corporate fashion. The National Advisory Commission on Health Facilities concluded as far back as 1968 that "the nation must now concentrate upon organizing health facilities and other health resources into effective, efficient, and economical community systems of comprehensive health-care available to all."[4]

ADAPTATION OF DISCIPLINES

The sociologist Eliot Freidson documents the tendency of the medical profession to expand its domain.[5] Physicians restructure disciplines and subspecialize to embrace newfound responsibilities; thus, for example, geriatrics is one of nine subspecialties and nine added qualifications of internal medicine. There is an alternative approach proposed in corporate America—adaptation of disciplines to the particular problems. The health professions have a better probability than single practitioners do of developing a strategy to address the problems of the geriatric population. The nursing model, with its functional strategies, can better meet the needs of the elderly than the medical model, with its exclusively curative focus, can. As exemplary geriatric programs in Edinburgh and Glasgow demonstrate, the movement from disciplinary to multidisciplinary to interdisciplinary approaches in collaborative practice need not reduce physician prerogatives or clinical authority.[6]

PROFESSIONAL EDUCATION AS A CONTINUUM

During the 1980s, AT&T, IBM, and General Motors each spent more on education and human-resource development annually than the combined educational budgets of the entire Ivy League.[7] The health labor force is eight times the combined employment of AT&T, IBM, and General Motors, yet the entire health-care enterprise does not invest as much in continuing education as any one of these companies does. The fact that health professionals are dispersed primarily in small institutions makes career development and the proliferation of continuing-education programs difficult. The increasing merger of institutions and the concentration of resources into larger delivery systems will both mandate and facilitate ongoing executive and professional development programs.

PHYSICIANS' PARTICIPATION AS CITIZENS

The surplus of approximately 145,000 physicians projected for the year 2000 could mean a larger number of physicians in positions of community leadership—that is, in parent-teacher associations; on church, synagogue, school, and charity boards; and in elective office. Their involvement at the community level will be crucial when, for example, school boards grapple with the problems of sex education, AIDS, substance abuse, and violence, or when communities seek to organize home-care hospice programs or when groups want to fund programs to respond to the needs of the homeless.

Physicians of my generation have characteristically worked sixty or more hours per week in their clinical practices. I anticipate that my students may work the same hours but devote more time to pro bono service to the community. That time will be the equivalent of the half-day or so per week donated by physicians to clinics and hospitals prior to the passage of Medicare and Medicaid. A reemergence of the eleemosynary convictions of medicine will benefit the profession as well as the community.

THE SYNTHESIS OF MEDICINE AND PUBLIC HEALTH

The passive strategy of the physician waiting in his or her office contrasts vividly with the activist strategy of the public-health professional working to launch immunization and cancer-screening programs, referendums on fluoridation, and occupational-health initiatives. Public health is based on principles that can be incorporated into medicine in a variety of ways. Medical practice quite properly focuses on advocacy for the individual patient; public health has accountability for a population. Whereas physicians have traditionally set both price and volume of service, public health requires resource allocation through prospective budgets. When, in the future, decisions on resource allocation are made, medicine can participate with public health or have the priorities set by others.

Formidable changes lie ahead. To those who are happy with the status quo and benefit from it, the changes may seem revolutionary. It is my conviction, though, that incrementalism will prevail in the American health-care enterprise.

Richard J. Franke, chairman and chief executive officer of John Nuveen, a company that underwrites and sells municipal bonds that fund the infrastructure of health-care systems, sums up the paradox of the enterprise when he says, "The irony of the health-care problem is that its foundations are rooted in the best-intentioned and sometimes contradictory principles the American society has developed and holds dear."[8] Americans' best intentions and contradictions are their strength as well as their weakness. And thus I look to the pluralism and pragmatism of health-care strategies to resolve the current paradox.

A pluralistic paradigm depends on the development of provider and consumer self-control. Moreover, it is imperative to maintain the flexibility and capacity to address problems not yet anticipated. The dozens upon dozens of biomedical advances of recent decades have radically altered needs, demands, issues, strategies, and responses in ways that no one could readily have predicted. That phenomenon is certain to intensify in the twenty-first century.

As I concluded a first draft of this chapter, the University of Pennsylvania celebrated the 250th anniversary of its founding by Benjamin Franklin in 1740, a half-century before ratification of the Bill of Rights. The university's motto, *Leges sine moribus vanae*—"Laws without values are meaningless"—applies to the present moment. The search for health security must reflect the society's values and its emerging conviction that health care is a right for all Americans.

Notes

Chapter 1. Somebody Has to Pay

1. Stephen E. Ambrose, *Eisenhower the President* (New York: Simon & Schuster, 1983), 271–72.
2. *Generally Speaking: Annual Report*, Lancaster General Hospital, 1990 91. Judge Bucher had open-heart surgery in 1973 and 1990. At Lancaster General Hospital, where more than 1,000 open-heart procedures were performed in 1989, a coronary artery bypass graft procedure with cardiac catheterization cost $23,000. The cost ranged up to $86,000 at other hospitals in the region.
3. Geert Meester and Francesco Pinciroli, eds., "Developments in Cardiovascular Medicine," *Databases for Cardiology* (Boston: Kluwer Academic Publishing, 1991).
4. James H. Cassedy, *Medicine in America: A Short History* (Baltimore: Johns Hopkins University Press, 1991), 141–42.
5. Steffie Woolhandler and David V. Himmelstein, "The Deteriorating Administrative Efficiency of the U.S. Health Care System," *New England Journal of Medicine*, 2 May 1991, 1253–58.

6. W. Williams, *America's First Hospital: The Pennsylvania* (Wayne, Pa.: Haverford House, 1976), 2–4, 8.
7. O. Anderson, *Blue Cross since 1929: Accountability and the Public Trust* (Cambridge: Ballinger Publishing Company, 1975), 18–19.
8. Rosemary Stevens, *In Sickness and in Wealth: American Hospitals in the Twentieth Century* (New York: Basic Books, 1989), 432.
9. Eliot Freidson, *Profession of Medicine: A Study of the Sociology of Applied Knowledge* (New York: Dodd, Mead, 1970), 409.
10. Suzanne W. Letsch et al., "National Health Expenditures," *Health Care Financing Review* 14, no. 2 (1992): 1–30.

Chapter 2. Health-Care Issues of the 1990s

1. Sir Geoffrey Vickers, "What Sets the Goals of Public Health?" *New England Journal of Medicine*, 20 March 1958, 589–96.
2. William L. Kissick, "The Pew Charitable Trusts and Health Policy: An Evaluation of Achievements and Opportunities" (report to the foundation, 21 December 1987).
3. Bureau of the Census, *Statistical Abstract of the United States, 1992*, 12th ed. (Washington, D.C.: GPO, 1992).
4. Linda Aiken and Claire Fagin, eds., "Strategies to Reduce Infant Mortality," *Charting Nursing's Future: Agenda for the Nineties* (Philadelphia: Lippincott, 1992), 304–05. Infant mortality has long been considered an accurate indicator of a community's and a nation's overall health.
5. Henry J. Aaron, Barry P. Bosworth, and Gary Burtless, *Can America Afford to Grow Old?* (Washington, D.C.: Brookings Institution, 1989), 144.
6. F. J. Hellinger, "The Lifetime Cost of Treating a Person with HIV," *Journal of the American Medical Association*, 28 July 1993, 474–78.
    There are approximately one million HIV-infected persons in the United States. The World Health Organization expects there to be 40 million HIV-infected individuals worldwide by 1995 (Antonia C. Novello, "The HIV/AIDS Epidemic: A Current Picture," *AIDS Research and Human Retroviruses* 8, no. 5 [1992]: 695–707.
7. H. W. Cushing, *The Life of Sir William Osler* (Oxford: Clarendon Press, 1925).
8. Kurt L. Schmoke, "Back to the Future: The Public Health System's Role in Fighting Drugs," *American Oxonian* 77, no. 1 [Winter 1990]: 1–9.
9. *Smoking and Health*, report of the Advisory Committee to the Surgeon

General, Public Health Service, Department of Health, Education, and Welfare (Washington, D.C.: GPO, 1964 and 1984).

10. *Physicians for a Growing America*, report of the Surgeon General's Consultant Group on Medical Education, Public Health Service, Department of Health, Education, and Welfare (Washington, D.C.: GPO, 1959); *Toward Quality in Nursing: Needs and Goals*, report of the Surgeon General's Consultant Group on Nursing, Public Health Service, Department of Health, Education, and Welfare (Washington, D.C.: GPO, 1963).

11. Report of the Graduate Medical Education National Advisory Committee to the Secretary, Department of Health and Human Services (Washington, D.C.: Health Resources Administration, Public Health Service, 1980).

12. Linda H. Aiken and Connie Flynt Mullinix, "The Nursing Shortage: Myth or Reality?" *New England Journal of Medicine*, 3 September 1987, 641–46.

13. Lisa F. Berkman and Lester Breslow, *Health and Ways of Living: The Alameda County Study* (New York: Oxford University Press, 1983), 237.

14. Eliot Freidson, *Patients' Views of Medical Practice* (Philadelphia: Russell Sage Foundation, 1961), 268.

15. James D. Lubitz and Gerald F. Riley, "Trends in Medicare Payments in the Last Year of Life," *New England Journal of Medicine*, 15 April 1993, 1093.

16. Derek Humphry, *Final Exit: The Practicalities of Self-Deliverance and Assisted Suicide for the Dying* (Eugene, Oreg.: Hemlock Society, 1991); Timothy Quill, "Death and Dignity: A Case of Individualized Decision Making," *New England Journal of Medicine*, 7 March 1991, 691–94.

17. President's Commission on Heart Disease, Cancer, and Stroke, *A National Program to Conquer Heart Disease, Cancer, and Stroke: Report to the President* (Washington, D.C.: GPO, 1964).

Chapter 3. An Infinite Quest

1. Edmund Jan Osmanozyla, *The Encyclopedia of the United Nations and International Relations* (New York: Taylor and Francis, 1990), 1035. WHO was established in 1948 as the central agency directing international health work. The definition appears in its constitution.

2. René Dubos, *Mirage of Health Utopias, Progress, and Biological Change* (Garden City, N.Y.: Doubleday, 1959), 1.

3. D. F. Sullivan, *Conceptual Problems in Developing an Index of Health*, Public Health Service Publication 1000, ser. 2, no. 17, 1966.

4. Public Information Office, Bureau of the Census, Washington, D.C.

5. *Origin, Program, and Operation of the U.S. National Health Survey,* National Center for Health Statistics, ser. 1, no. 1, August 1963.

6. The goals were (1) "to continue to improve infant health, and, by 1990, to reduce infant mortality by at least 35 percent, to fewer than nine deaths per 1,000 live births"; (2) "to improve child health, foster optimal childhood development, and, by 1990, reduce deaths among children ages one to 14 years by at least 20 percent, to fewer than 34 per 100,000"; (3) "to improve the health and health habits of adolescents and young adults, and, by 1990, to reduce deaths among people ages 15 to 24 by at least 20 percent, to fewer than 93 per 100,000"; (4) "improve the health of adults, and, by 1990, to reduce deaths among people ages 25 to 64 by at least 25 percent, to fewer than 400 per 100,000"; and (5) "to improve the health and quality of life for older adults, and, by 1990, to reduce the average annual number of days of restricted activity due to acute and chronic conditions by 20 percent, to fewer than 30 days per year for people aged 65 and older" (Public Health Service, Department of Health, Education, and Welfare, *Healthy People: The Surgeon General's Report on Health Promotion and Disease Prevention* [Washington, D.C.: GPO, 1979], 177). The Year 2000 Health Objectives Planning Act of 1990 established grants to help states develop plans for improving the health status of their populations. It also called for the establishment of a uniform set of health-status indicators for use by federal, state, and local agencies.

7. "Health Objectives for the Nation: Consensus Set of Health Status Indicators for the General Assessment of Community Health Status— United States," *Morbidity and Mortality Weekly Report,* 12 July 1991.

Chapter 4. A Cultural Affair

1. Derek Gill, *The British National Health Service: A Sociologist's Perspective* (Washington, D.C.: Department of Health and Human Services, 1980). The Health Insurance Act of 1911 provided a limited degree of medical care to people who fell into specific occupational and financial categories. It entitled them to free treatment and care by general practitioners.

2. Department of Health and Social Security, *Management Arrangements for the Reorganized National Health Service* (London: HMSO, 1972); *The NHS Reorganization* (London: Office of Health Economics, 1974).

3. Clifford Graham, "Listen to the Individual Person: A Human Response to the Health and Social Services Consumer" (Department of Health and Social Security, 1990, photocopy).

4. Royal Commission on Health Services, *Report* (Ottawa: Queen's Printer, 1964).

5. *Canadian Health Care: The Implications of Public Health Insurance*, research bulletin of the Health Insurance Association of America, June 1990, 100; T. Marmor, "Commentary on Canadian Health Insurance: Lessons for the United States," *International Journal of Health Services* 23, no. 1 (1993): 45–62.

6. Abraham Flexner, *Medical Education in the United States and Canada* (New York: Carnegie Foundation, 1910), 346.

7. Ministry of Health, Consultative Council on Medical and Allied Service, *Interim Report on the Future Provision of Medical and Allied Services* (London: HMSO, 1920).

8. Alain C. Enthoven, "Reflections on the Management of the National Health Service: An American Looks at Incentives to Efficiency in Health Services Management in the U.K." Nuffield Provincial Hospitals Trust Occasional Papers 5, London, 1985.

Chapter 5. Resource Allocation

1. Organization for Economic Cooperation and Development, *Health Systems, Facts, and Trends, 1990–1991*, Paris, 1993, 1:08–09.

2. Adam Smith contends that markets work without interference, as if guided by an "invisible hand," to ensure the most efficient allocation of resources (*An Inquiry into the Nature and Causes of the Wealth of Nations* [Oxford: Clarendon Press, 1976]; see also his *Theory of Moral Sentiment* [Oxford: Clarendon Press, 1976]).

3. Paul A. Samuelson and William D. Nordhaus *Economics* (New York: McGraw-Hill, 1992), 784.

4. Eugene G. McCarthy and Geraldine W. Widmer, "Effects of Screening by Consultants on Recommended Elective Surgical Procedures," *New England Journal of Medicine*, 19 December 1974, 1331–35.

5. John D. Thompson, "On Reasonable Costs of Hospital Services," part 2, *Dimensions and Determinants of Health Policy* 46, no. 1 (1968): 33–51.

6. Department of Health and Human Services, Public Health Service, Agency for Health Care Policy and Research, *Acute Pain Management:*

Operative or Medical Procedures and Trauma (Washington, D.C.: GPO, 1992), 145.

7. James D. Lubitz and Gerald F. Riley, "Trends in Medicare Payments in the Last Year of Life," *New England Journal of Medicine*, 15 April 1993, 1093.

8. Anne R. Somers and Nancy L. Spears, *The Continuing Care Retirement Community: A Significant Option for Long-Term Care* (New York: Springer, 1992), 206.

9. S. T. Sonnefeld et al., "Projections for Health Expenditures through the Year 2000," *Health Care Financing Review* 13 (fall 1991): 1–38.

10. A. Laupacis et al., "The Cost-Effectiveness of Routine Post Myocardial Infarction Exercise Stress Testing," *Canadian Journal of Cardiology* 6, no. 4 (1990): 157–63; T. Byers and R. Gorsky, "Estimates of Costs and Effects of Screening for Colorectal Cancer in the United States," *Cancer* 70, no. 5 supplement (1992): 1288–95.

11. J. E. Wennberg, "Future Directions for Small Area Variations," *Medical Care* 31, no. 5 supplement (1993): 75–80; Wennberg, "Geographic Variations in Expenditures for Physicians' Services in the United States," *New England Journal of Medicine*, 4 March 1993, 621–27; Wennberg, "Dealing with Geographic Variations in the Use of Hospitals," *Journal of Bone and Joint Surgery* 72, no. 9 (1990): 1286–93.

12. *Annual Report, 1992*, Group Health Cooperative of Puget Sound, 521 Wall St., Seattle, Wash. 98121. Facts are updated to May 1993.

Chapter 6. Medicine and Management

1. William L. Kissick, "Health Care Management according to Ben Franklin," *Journal of health Administration Education* 7, no. 4 (1989): 723–33.

2. Paul Starr, *The Social Transformation of American Medicine: The Rise of a Sovereign Profession and the Making of a Vast Industry* (New York: Basic Books, 1982), 420–49; Arnold S. Relman, "The New Medical-Industrial Complex," *New England Journal of Medicine*, 23 October 1980, 963–70.

3. Gunnar Myrdal, *Beyond the Welfare State: Economic Planning and Its International Implications* (New Haven: Yale University Press, 1960), 47.

4. Andrew A. Skolnick, "Joint Commission Will Collect, Publicize Outcomes," *Journal of the American Medical Association*, 14 July 1993, 165, 168, 171; M. Roy Schwarz, "Liaison Committee on Medical Education: Past Successes, Future Challenges," *Journal of the American Medical Association*, 2 September 1992, 1091–92.

Chapter 7. The Past as Prologue

1. Charles S. Lindblom, *The Policy-Making Process* (Englewood Cliffs: Prentice-Hall), 1980, and "The Science of Muddling Through," *Public Administration Review* 19 (1959): 79–88. Lindblom advances the concept of disjointed, or fragmented, incrementalism to characterize the evolution of social policy.

2. Beverlee A. Myers, *Concepts and Principles*, vol. 1 of *Guide to Medical Care Administration* (New York: American Public Health Association, 1965), appendix 3. This chronology traces almost 150 private- and public-sector health initiatives from colonial times to the late twentieth century.

3. *Medical Care for the American People· Final Report of the Committee on the Costs of Medical Care* (Chicago: University of Chicago Press, 1932), 223.

4. The Committee on Economic Security, appointed by President Roosevelt in 1934 to devise plans for a Social Security system, recommended "federal pensions, unemployment insurance and direct assistance for certain categories of the needy, and suggested that an official study be made on the practicability of national health insurance" (Richard Harris, *A Sacred Trust* [New York: Penguin, 1966], 8–9).

5. Federal Works Agency, Work Projects Administration, *Final Statistical Report of the Federal Emergency Relief Association* (Washington, D.C.: GPO, 1942), iii.

6. House Committee on Ways and Means, *Economic Security Act: Hearings on H.R. 4120*, 74th Cong., 1st sess., 1935, 1141; Senate Committee on Finance, *Economic Security Act: Hearings on S.R. 1130*, 74th Cong., 1st sess., 1935, 1354.

7. Myers, *Concepts and Principles*, appendix 3.

8. Harris, *A Sacred Trust*, 280. The Wagner-Murray-Dingell bill, providing compulsory national health insurance for employees and their dependents, included physicians' services, hospitalization, diagnostic services, and drugs. Financing was based on employer and employee contributions and was to be administered through the states. The bill never made it to the floor of the House or Senate.

9. The Hill-Burton program was named for its sponsors, Senator Lister Hill of Alabama and Representative Charles Burton of Ohio. It authorized investments of federal tax dollars in the construction of hospitals, with initial priority given to rural areas. During its almost three decades, some $20 billion of federal funds were invested through grants-in-aid to community, public, and not-for-profit health-care facilities.

10. Oscar R. Ewing, *The Nation's Health: A Ten-Year Program. A Report to the President* (Washington, D.C.: GPO, 1948), 186.

11. Stephen P. Strickland, *Politics, Science, and Dread Disease: A Short History of United States Medical Research Policy* (Cambridge: Harvard University Press, 1972), 329; Zoe E. Boniface and Rebecca W. Rimel, *U.S. Funding for Biomedical Research* (Philadelphia: Pew Charitable Trusts, 1987), 85.

12. J. W. Mountin, E. H. Pennell, and V. M. Hoge, *Health Service Areas: Requirements for General Hospitals and Health Centers*, Public Health Service Publication 292 (Washington: GPO, 1945). This classic study of regional planning was carried out in the Office of the Surgeon General during World War II. Every county was allocated to a primary or secondary service area for referral of patients from community health centers to regional specialized centers. The document, which drew on Lord Dawson's 1923 *Report on Regionalization of Health Services in the United Kingdom*, served as the basic staff work for the Hill-Burton program and contributed conceptually to the regional medical programs of 1965.

13. William L. Kissick, "Health Manpower in Transition," *Dimensions and Determinants of Health Policy*, January 1968, 53–90.

14. *Physicians for a Growing America*, report of the Surgeon General's Consultant Group on Medical Education, Public Health Service, Department of Health, Education, and Welfare (Washington, D.C.: GPO, 1959). The report recommended producing, by 1970, as many more graduates as would be turned out by twenty new medical schools. The Health Professions Education Assistance Act of 1963 was drafted to implement the recommendations of the report.

15. Public Health Service, report of the Surgeon General's Consultant Group on Nursing, *Toward Quality in Nursing: Needs and Goals*, Department of Health, Education, and Welfare (Washington, D.C.: GPO, 1963).

16. William L. Kissick, "Health Policy Directions for the 1970's," *New England Journal of Medicine*, 11 June 1970, 1343–54.

17. The Comprehensive Health Planning and Public Health Service Amendments of 1966, known as the Partnership for Health, encompassed three legislative strategies in one: (1) health planning that attempted to generalize area-wide hospital planning to the full spectrum of health concerns, (2) formula or block grants to the states to fund public-health services that could be traced back to Title VI of the Social Security Act of 1935, and (3) project grants for health-services demon-

strations to provide seed money for designing and launching innovative comprehensive health-care systems.

18. Lawrence P. Brown, *Politics and Health Care Organization: HMOs as Federal Policy* (Washington, D.C.: Brookings Institution, 1983), 540.

Chapter 8. National Health Insurance

1. David V. Himmelstein and Steffie Woolhandler, "A National Health Program for the United States: A Physician's Proposal," *New England Journal of Medicine*, 12 January 1989, 102–07.

2. Mark V. Pauly et al., *Responsible National Health Insurance* (Washington, D.C.: American Enterprise Institute, 1992), 87.

3. Robert D. Eilers, "National Health Insurance: What Kind and How Much?" *New England Journal of Medicine*, 22 April 1971, 881–86; 29 April 1971, 945–54; Marcia Angell, "The Presidential Candidates and Health Care Reform," *New England Journal of Medicine*, 10 September 1992, 800–01.

4. Alain C. Enthoven, "Consumer-Choice Health Plan," *New England Journal of Medicine*, 23 March 1978, 650–58; 30 March 1978, 709–20; 5 January 1989, 29–37; 12 January 1989, 94–101. See also Enthoven, "Shattuck Lecture: Cutting Cost without Cutting the Quality of Care," *New England Journal of Medicine*, 1 June 1978, 1229–38, and *Health Plan: The Only Practical Solution to the Soaring Cost of Medical Care* (Reading, Mass.: Addison-Wesley, 1980), 196.

Chapter 9. "To the States Respectively"

1. A good clinician is concerned about potential side effects of therapeutic strategies. The physician shortage of the 1960s became the surplus of the 1980s as a consequence of medical school expansion, immigration of foreign-trained physicians, creation of off-shore schools of medicine, and erroneous population projections for determining needs. Medicare's adoption of open-ended financing resulted in inflation and increased utilization. Student loans have enabled young physicians to start careers with debts of $150,000 and more.

2. Beverlee A. Myers, *Concepts and Principles*, vol. 1 of *Guide to Medical Care Administration* (New York: American Public Health Association, 1965), appendix 3.

3. Marcus Rosenblum, ed., *Compendium on Workmen's Compensation* (Washington, D.C.: GPO, 1973), 16. The workers' compensation law imple-

mented in Wisconsin in 1911 was the first such law to "become and remain effective." Protection was not provided in every state until 1948.

4. Paul Starr, *The Social Transformation of American Medicine: The Rise of a Sovereign Profession and the Making of a Vast Industry* (New York: Basic Books, 1982), 514.

5. Joseph P. Anderson, "Arizona Health Care Cost-Containment," *Journal of the Florida Medical Association* 73, no. 2 (1987): 106–09.

6. Howard E. Freeman and Bradford L. Kirkman-Liff, "Health Care under AHCCCS: An Examination of Arizona's Alternative to Medicaid," *Health Services Research* 20, no. 3 (1985): 247.

7. Deane Neubauer, "Hawaii: A Pioneer in Health System Reform," *Health Affairs* 12, no. 2 (1993): 32.

8. CHAMPUS provides financial coverage of health-care services for military personnel and their families when they use nonmilitary health facilities. Because of the large concentration of military personnel (a quarter of the population), CHAMPUS plays a unique role in Hawaii.

9. Eleanor D. Kinney and William P. Gronfein, "Indiana's Malpractice System: No-Fault by Accident?" *Law & Contemporary Problems* 54, no. 1 (1991): 169–93.

10. Larry S. Milner, "The Constitutionality of Medical Malpractice Legislative Reform: A National Survey," *Loyola University of Chicago Law Journal* 18, no. 3 (1987): 1053–84.

11. Roger L. Williams, *The Origins of Federal Support for Higher Education: George W. Atherton and the Land-Grant College Movement* (University Park: Pennsylvania State University Press, 1991), 12. The Morrill Act provided an indirect endowment to support at least one college per state whose main focus was to be on "such branches of learning as are related to agriculture and the mechanic arts." The act is viewed as marking the beginning of federal involvement in higher education.

12. *Ninety-two Years of Serving Iowans*, University of Iowa Hospital and Clinics Service Record, 1989–90, exhibits 1–2, 1990.

13. William L. Kissick, "Regional Medical Programs," *Northwest Medicine* 64 (December 1965): 971–79.

14. Gerard Anderson, Patrick Chaulk, and Elizabeth Fowler, "Maryland: A Regulatory Approach to Health System Reform," *Health Affairs* 12, no. 2 (1993): 41.

15. Karen Davis et al., *Health Care Cost-Containment* (Baltimore: Johns Hopkins University Press, 1990), 35.

16. Alan Sager, Deborah Socolar, and Peter Hjam. "Nine Lessons for National Health Reform from the Failure of the 1988 Massachusetts Uni-

versal Health Insurance Law." American Public Health Association, 26 October 1993. Unpublished ms.

17. R. L. Reece, "The Corporate Transformation of Medicine in Minnesota: The Grand Finale and the Grand Finesse," *Minnesota Medicine*, November 1987, 609–13; B. A. Elliott, "State 'Laboratories' Test Health Care Reform Solution," *Minnesota Medicine*, February 1993, 14–21.

18. Christine M. Grant, senior director of public policy, Merck & Company, Inc., personal communication.

19. Department of Labor, Labor-Management Services Administration, *Employee Retirement Income Security Act*, 1975 Report to Congress, 1–3. ERISA, signed into law in 1974 by President Gerald R. Ford, was designed to protect workers who participate in private pension and welfare plans, as well as their beneficiaries.

20. Harvey D. Klevit et al., "Prioritization of Health Care Services: A Progress Report by the Oregon Health Services Commission," *Archives of Internal Medicine* 151 (May 1991): 912. Although Coby Howard became a symbol for those opposed to the legislation, supporters pointed out that the boy was not in remission and thus not a good candidate for bone-marrow transplantation.

21. Uwe E. Reinhardt, "Health Insurance for the Nation's Poor," *Health Affairs* 6, no. 1 (1987): 101–12.

22. Jennifer Dixon and H. Gilbert Welch, "Priority Setting: Lessons from Oregon," *Lancet*, 23 April 1991, 891. Recognizing the confusion surrounding the Coby Howard case, Kitzhaber, an emergency-room physician, based the Oregon plan on development of a health-service priority ranking to "ensure that the distribution of public dollars would be made more rationally and openly."

23. "Overview, Health Services Act of 1993" (Health Care Authority, State of Washington, May 1993, photocopy), 33.

24. Robert A. Crittenden, "Managed Competition and Premium Caps in Washington State," *Health Affairs* 12, no. 2 (1993): 82–88.

Chapter 10. Promoting the General Welfare

1. John R. Lott, "Why Is Education Publicly Provided? A Critical Survey," *Cato Journal* 7, no. 2 (1987): 475–97.

2. Henry Aaron, *Serious and Unstable Condition: Financing America's Health Care* (Washington, D.C.: Brookings Institution, 1991), 64. Federal guidelines help determine how Medicaid pays for acute and long-term

care in individual states; eligibility criteria and benefits vary greatly from state to state.

3. As of 1990, V.A. facilities included 172 hospitals, 32 domiciliaries, 226 outpatient clinics, and 126 nursing homes; 1,113,000 inpatients were treated, and there were 22.6 million outpatient visits (*Annual Report of the Secretary of Veterans Affairs: Directory of V.A. Facilities*, 1990). In 1991, approximately $12.6 billion was spent on the hospital and medical care of veterans (Health Care Financing Administration, *Health Care Financing Review*, fall 1992).

4. Lisbeth B. Schorr, "Reforming National Health Policies," *Within Our Reach: Breaking the Cycle of Disadvantage* (New York: Doubleday, 1988), 111–39.

5. Edward Zigler and Sally Styfco, eds., *Head Start and Beyond* (New Haven: Yale University Press, 1993). Project Head Start, born in the 1960s, reflects the belief that education is the solution to poverty and other social ills. Launched to provide services to prepare low-income preschoolers for elementary school, it led to the formation of other federal programs to assist children through their school years.

6. David W. Sayen, Staff Assistant, Region III, Health Care Financing Administration, U.S. Department of Health and Human Services, personal communication.

7. Karl Schriftgeiser, *Business Comes of Age: The Story of the Committee for Economic Development and Its Impact upon the Economic Policies of the United States, 1942–1960* (New York: Harper Brothers, 1961), 5.

8. Steven Bailey, *Congress Makes a Law: The Story behind the Employment Act of 1946* (New York: Random House, 1974).

Chapter 11. Hang Together or Hang Separately

1. A preferred provider organization is a group of providers that contracts with a third-party payer, self-insured industry, or union trust fund to sell health services to a defined group of patients at preferential fee-for-service rates. A PPO may be a group of physicians, a hospital, or other organization. It lowers charges in return for prompt payment, regular volume, and the inherent competitive advantage. Insured individuals may see the doctors of their choice, but they forfeit first-dollar coverage and face cost sharing if they do not use PPO services (Lee Hyde, *Essential Dictionary of Health Care: A Practical Reference for Physicians and Nurses* [New York: McGraw-Hill, 1988], 348).

2. An independent practice association is a legal entity that has entered into an arrangement with providers, a majority of whom are licensed to

practice medicine or osteopathy. The IPA may be a partnership, a corporation, or any other legal entity. The arrangement between it and the providers require that they provide their professional services in accordance with its compensation plan. The term originated, and is defined, in the Health Maintenance Organization Act of 1974. IPAS are one source of professional services for health maintenance organizations and are modeled after medical foundations (Hyde, 264).

3. Ray E. Brown, personal communication. Brown was one of the eight members of the White House task force appointed by President Johnson to make recommendations for the Great Society's health program. As vice president of the University of Chicago Medical Center, he argued for the imperatives of options and choices

4. Warren H. Schmidt and Jerome P. Finnigan, *The Race without a Finish Line: America's Quest for Total Quality* (San Francisco: Jossey-Bass, 1992), 402. Total quality management involves (1) customer satisfaction, (2) challenge (establishing clear, challenging, but achievable goals), (3) processing and planning (developing a well-defined process to achieve goals), (4) continuous improvement, (5) collaboration within organizations, (6) change, (7) measurement, and (8) persistence.

5. H. Darlene Burgess, vice president for corporate government relations, Henry Ford Health System, personal communication.

6. Wanda A. Current, Public Relations Department, Group Health Cooperative, personal communication.

7. Carole Welch, Public and Community Relations Department, Central Office, Kaiser Permanente, personal communication.

8. Jake Getson, Officer, U.S. Healthcare, personal communication.

9. Bruce W. Herdman, Vice President, Medical Delivery, Keystone Health Plan East, personal communication.

10. Draft Proceedings, Regional Medical Programs: Twenty-fifth-Anniversary Conference, 6 December 991, National Library of Medicine, Bethesda, Md.

Chapter 12. Health Care for the Twenty-first Century

1. *The President's Health Security Plan* (New York: Times Books/Random House, 1993).

2. Myron Fottler et al., "Public Release of Hospital-Specific Death Rates: Guidelines for Health Care Executives," *Hospital and Health Services Administration*, August 1987, 343–56. Changes in the regulatory guidelines of the Freedom of Information Act have allowed greater public access to hospital-specific data on Medicare patients. The effect has been a sub-

stantial increase in media attention to hospital outcomes, especially death rates.

3. Avi Dor, Philip J. Held, and Mark V. Pauly, "The Medical Cost of Renal Dialysis," *Medical Care* 30, no. 10 (1992): 878–91. Medicare's costs are more than $6 billion per year for renal dialysis, kidney transplants, and other lifesaving measures for 190,000 patients.

4. National Advisory Commission on Health Facilities, *Report to the President*, 12 December 1968, 6. The commission was appointed by President Johnson to evaluate the role of the Hill-Burton program in the development and provision of health services.

5. Eliot Freidson, *Profession of Medicine: A Study of the Sociology of Applied Knowledge* (New York: Dodd, Mead, 1970).

6. Sir Ferguson Anderson and Brian Williams, "Organization of a Geriatric Service," *Practical Management of the Elderly*, 5th ed. (Oxford: Blackwell Scientific, 1989), 327–53; Neville E. Strumpf, associate professor of nursing, University of Pennsylvania, personal communication.

7. Robert M. Zemsky, professor of education and director, Institute of Research in Higher Education, University of Pennsylvania, personal communication; Martin Myerson, president emeritus, University of Pennsylvania, personal communication.

8. Richard J. Franke, "Resolving the Health-Care Paradox: A Need for National Debate" (Robert D. Eilers Memorial Lecture, University of Pennsylvania, 1990), 15.

Index

175

physicians (continued)
66–68; new roles for, 71, 84,
158–59
Physicians Desk Reference (PDR), 26
Physicians for a Growing America, 79–
80
Pillsbury corporation, 111
"play or pay" strategy, 87, 89–90,
91, 93–94, 110
pluralism, 64, 72–73, 151, 159–60
policy institutes, 40, 41
polio vaccine, 5–6, 155
poor citizens, 32, 82, 89, 90, 91,
110, 116
population factors, 75, 77–78, 133,
137
preexisting conditions, 116
preferred provider organizations
(PPOS), 43, 134–35, 138, 172n1
prenatal care, 32, 59, 60, 114
prepaid health plan, 96, 103, 137
prescription medications, 12, 14–
15, 103, 127, 128, 129, 154–55
President's Commission on Heart
Disease, Cancer and Stroke, 22
President's Health Security Plan, 149,
154
prevention of disease, 15, 20, 25,
59–60, 126
primary care, 26, 27, 145–48
prior authorization, 55, 143
private sector, 72–73, 90
"professional liability insurance,"
12, 19
professional standards review organizations (PSROS), 83
provider associations, 40–41, 52
Prudential, 41, 72
public assistance, 80–81, 96
public health, 29, 34–35, 79, 159
public sector, 86–87

quality health care, 2–3, 38, 92, 93,
94, 138–39, 149
quality of life, 22, 155
"queuing," 42, 62
Quill, Timothy, 21

RAND corporation, 40
Ru-486, 16
rate-setting, 108–09
rationing, 58, 61–62, 71, 129, 138,
156–57
Reagan administration, xiv
reform in health care, 79, 86–87,
98–100, 117; countries compared,
45–47; principles, 135–38, 149–
50; prototypes for, 139–42; management of, 142–45; legislation,
151–53; factors in, 154–60
regional programs, 147, 151
religious institutions, 43, 71
Relman, Arnold S., 69
renal dialysis, 4, 5–6, 63, 155
*Report on Health Promotion and Disease
Prevention*, 31
research, 40, 78–79
Residual Malpractice Insurance Authority, 106
resource allocation, 71, 156–57. *See
also* financing health care
resource-based/relative-value scales,
56, 72, 73, 84, 144
retrospective cost-based reimbursement, 10, 70
right to die, 20–22
right to health care, 8, 39, 118–19,
120–21
Rockefeller, John D., IV, 89
Röntgen, Wilhelm Konrad, 4
Roosevelt, Franklin D., 77
Royal Commission on Health Services, 37

St. Louis Park Medical Center, 110
San Joaquin Medical Care Foundation, 141
Saskatchewan, 36, 37
Schmoke, Kurt L., 17
Scots Charitable Society, 109
second opinion, 55, 143–44
Senate-House health committee, 153
sex education, 13–14
Silber, John, 21
single payer strategy, 87–89, 91, 93
small businesses, 90, 91, 99, 104, 105, 116, 127
Smith, Adam, 165*n*2
Social Security, 49, 121; Act, 77, 79, 102; amendments, 81, 83
Social Transformation of American Medicine (Starr), 69
solo practice, 9, 34, 43, 81, 82, 88, 135, 137–38
special interest groups, 87
specialization, 17–18, 26, 27–28, 42, 67, 70, 157–58
"stakeholders," 70–71, 88, 153
Standard Hospital Accounting and Rate Evaluation, 112
Stark, Fortney, 98
Starr, Paul, 69
states' role in health care, 90, 99, 101–02, 117, 164*n*6. *See also* federal-state partnership
Straub Clinic, 104
strike, physicians', 37
stroke, 22, 59
Strumpf, Neville E., 174*n*6
substance abuse, 16–17, 102
surgical procedures, 9, 61, 120
Sweden, 48, 49, 58

tax legislation, 3–4, 48–49, 86–87, 88, 98, 100
technology, 24, 79, 145–46
teenage pregnancy, 13, 14, 125, 126
Terry, Luther L., 17
tertiary care, 26, 27, 145–48
therapeutic protocols, 57, 144
third-party insurance, 8, 10, 49, 50
tort reform, 19–20, 105–07
total quality management (TQM), 97, 139, 144, 173*n*4
trade-offs, 4, 97, 109, 150
Tripler Army Hospital, 104
Truman, Harry S., 38, 78

uninsured citizens, 3, 104, 111, 113, 115
United Auto Workers, 41
United Kingdom, 38, 39, 41–47. *See also* British National Health Service
United States, 31–32, 38–40; systems compared, 41–47; priorities in, 121–23
U.S. Healthcare, 141–42
U.S. Public Health Service, 25–26
U.S. Steel, xv
universal access, 58, 105, 110, 123; as goal, 91–92, 93, 94, 129–32, 149, 153–54
University of Connecticut, 147
University of Iowa, 107–08, 146, 147
University of Missouri, 147
University of Pennsylvania, 148
utilization review, 55, 144

Value for Money in Health (Abel-Smith), 13
Vermont, 152